THE
CHANGING
YEARS

Also by Madeline Gray

THE NORMAL WOMAN
MARGARET SANGER: A Biography of the Champion of Birth
Control

Madeline Gray

THE
CHANGING
YEARS

The Menopause Without Fear

THIRD REVISED EDITION

1981
Doubleday & Company, Inc.
Garden City, New York

Library of Congress Cataloging in Publication Data

Gray, Madeline.
The changing years.

Bibliography: p. 253
Includes index.
1. Menopause. I. Title. [DNLM: 1. Menopause—
Popular works. WP 580 G781c]
RG186.G7   1981   618.1'75
Library of Congress Catalog Card Number 77–16917
ISBN: 0-385-12635-2

Third Revised Edition

Contents

THE
CHANGING
YEARS

1

Somebody to Talk To

You're in your fifties, your forties, or even your thirties, and you're worried. For strange things have begun to happen to you.

You woke up with a start the other night, perhaps out of a deep, sound sleep. A great wave of heat was spreading from the tips of your breasts to the top of your head, drenching your nightgown and making you run to open the windows wide.

Or you have been having headaches. Not the old kind of headaches a couple of aspirin used to chase, but nauseating "sick" headaches with pain so intense your footsteps seem to echo as you walk from the bedroom to the bathroom door.

Or there have been days when your heart beat so loudly it seemed the whole world could hear it. Or other days when you were so inexplicably tired you could hardly drag yourself to the grocery store four blocks away.

Meanwhile that old business of menstruation has been acting up also—either skipping a month or arriving like a flood.

And what has been happening to your private world where everything had been so comparatively serene? The other day, for instance, you cuffed your daughter hard in an outburst of temper when she did something you'd been amused at the day before. The same evening at dinner you got furious at your husband for smacking his lips over his pork chops when for years you rather laughed at the habit, saying it proved he enjoyed your cooking. And to top it all you'd bawled like a baby when your son, to whom you'd said for months, "Isn't it about time you settled

down and got married?" came home and announced he'd gotten
the girl of his choice to say yes.

Why the strange physical upsets? Why the even stranger
emotional ones?

Gradually it dawns on you: This is it! The menopause, the
dreaded "change of life." It is happening to you at last.

As a result, you may be quite worried by the situation—not
so much by one thing as by the whole picture. A few passing
aches and pains you can take in your stride. But suppose it adds
up to permanent trouble? Loss of energy forever? Temper out-
bursts indefinitely? Maybe also loss of your figure, loss of your
sex life, loss of your husband's love, loss of your mind? All the
old fears drawn from centuries of gossip and ignorance crowd in
upon you. The picture looks dark indeed.

Well, you're not the only one to feel this way.

Every year millions of women are in the same condition as
you are—faced with what you are facing, asking the same questions that are tormenting you.

I asked myself the same questions. In fact, that's how I happened to write this book.

At the age of forty-six I had what is known as a surgical
menopause—a change brought on by a hysterectomy. That means
I was thrown into the midst of this thing headlong. I had no time
to get mentally set. And as I lay in my hospital bed all the old
fears crowded in on me. What was I in for? What would happen
to me? I was afraid I'd grow a mustache and gain forty pounds
at the very least. But really I hadn't the faintest idea.

The first chance I got, I cornered my surgeon and plied him
with questions. But while he was a distinguished man, and had
done an excellent job, he was too busy and too abrupt to bother
with me. He answered curtly that he'd done what he had to do
(which was far more than I had expected), and that was that. He
told me to go home and forget about the whole thing. Besides,
my pains were all imaginary.

This got me twice as worried as before. As if one could forget what one didn't understand! As if there is such a thing as an
"imaginary" pain! A pain is a pain. It may have an emotional
rather than a physical origin—that is, be caused by fear or mis-

understanding and so originate mainly in the mind. But that doesn't make it "imaginary" in the sense that you think you have a pain when you haven't. When you have a pain, you *have* one. And I had several at that moment, believe me.

So, with my surgeon ruled out as a source of information, I next tried questioning friends of my own age. But they knew less than I did. Worse, they knew all the horror stories. "You know Sarah Y down the block?" they asked in a hushed whisper. "*She* went out of her mind during her menopause. Yes, positively out!" Or: "I hear Mary G lost her husband Tom to another woman. And you could hardly blame Tom. After all, poor Mary had become quite hopeless in the realm of sex." Or: "Remember old lady Brown? She got both high blood pressure and arthritis during her change, and never was the same again."

My friends may have enjoyed telling me these juicy tales. But they hardly improved my peace of mind.

So next I tried speaking to some women who had gone through the menopause. Alas! The results were no better than before. Some also harped on the theme that "all the troubles are imaginary." This seemed to be because they themselves had had no trouble, which is, of course, often the case. And some went to the other extreme and boasted how they had been tortured for years. While still others actually told me to *expect* suffering "because suffering is the badge of all women." Didn't the Bible say, "In sorrow thou shalt bring forth children?" And didn't that apply to the menopause as well?

Next I looked for books that might help me. But there were almost none that satisfactorily answered all my questions.

Finally, I decided there was no other solution: I was a writer and former teacher; I would have to do a book myself. I was right in the midst of the experience; if I could learn the truth about menopause it would solve my own problems and maybe help others as well.

Yet the job wasn't going to be easy. It would mean talking to dozens and dozens of doctors—not only surgeons, but internists, hormone specialists, psychiatrists; and not only in the United States but also in Europe, wherever knowledge was to be found. Tracking down the whole elusive subject the way a detective tracks down clues. Especially it would mean tracking down the answer to the most haunting question of all: Why does a woman get *over* her menopausal troubles if she has any? What makes the adjustment? Why does she come out at the other end of the experience practically as good as she went in?

So I started. I worked at the New York Academy of Medicine; I traveled around the country; I spent hours in clinics talking to patients and doctors. And I wrote letters, letters, and more letters. Hardly a morning went by without my eagerly hopping out of bed to see what answers the mail had brought.

At last, after four years, I was through. Through with my search and through with my menopause. And during those four years, I found out the great principle at work within us—the "wisdom of the body" which brings us back to ourselves. I found that we do not lose our sex lives, lose our figures, lose our husbands, or our minds.

And as I found out these things, knowledge cast out my fears. Even on my darkest menopausal days (and having had a surgical menopause some of those days were dark indeed) I was optimistic. Not with the silly optimism of a Pollyanna, but an optimism based on fact.

I learned, for example, that prolonged suffering is unnecessary, since there is now, for the first time in history, blessed menopausal medicine to help. Our mothers may have had to suffer; not us. We are almost the first generation lucky enough to have this help.

I learned how to answer the people who quoted the Bible saying we *must* suffer and not use menopausal medicine. For the same people had used the Bible against the introduction of anesthesia in childbirth—used it until a witty Scots doctor answered them with an equally good Biblical quotation: "And the Lord caused a deep sleep to fall up Adam, and in that sleep brought forth Eve." Deep sleep is the best anesthetic in the world, the learned doctor pointed out; surely the Lord intended people to have relief from pain. So the skeptics should have been silenced once and for all, though it still took Queen Victoria, using anesthesia for the birth of her seventh child, to make it fashionable, so fashionable that it was known for a long time as "the anesthesia of the Queen."

But most important, I learned why menopausal medicine is often not needed, for the simple reason that no menopausal trouble occurs.

For the menopause is merely another step in life's dance. It is not a disease, and brings with it no disease. As a result, many of us take this step so comfortably we need no help. Our own "wisdom of the body" sees us through.

Having learned this, then, I began to write my book and share my knowledge—write it as if I were sitting down and talking to you in a peaceful chat. I decided to leave out nothing—touch on the hush-hush matters equally with the obvious matters —try to answer every last old wives' tale.

When you have finished reading it, I humbly believe that, instead of asking advice from your friends, you should be able to give it. Instead of pestering your mother, you should be able to enlighten her. And instead of arguing with your know-it-all husband, you should (oh, blessed state of affairs) be able to tell him a few things, too.

Since the original publication of *The Changing Years* I have received hundreds and hundreds of grateful letters. Encouraged by this enthusiastic reception I continued carefully to study the subject, and found that both the attitudes toward it and the treatment of it were in many ways different from before.

However, many of the old fears remained, and new ones even were added. There has been so much publicity on the relation of estrogen to cancer that women like my own sister refused to take the hormones they badly needed. So much discussion on the so-called male menopause that men were sure all of them, too, were in for a terrible time. So many questions about entering or re-entering the job market at mid-life, that a whole series of counseling sessions were devoted to it. And, because Americans have become more sex-conscious and weight-conscious than ever, fear to the point of panic that total loss of attractiveness was sure to arrive with the later years.

Yet, after years of personal experience and interviews with

many women and doctors, I still believe, as I write this revised edition, that the fears are greatly exaggerated.

The latter years can be full of hope instead of despair. For women especially, they can be a truly happy time.

2

Not *The Change* but *Another* Change

Once in the long ago someone did women a terrible injustice; in fact, it was one of the worst injustices ever done. This was the invention of a phrase to describe the menopause—a dreadful phrase that has wrought as much harm as all the horror stories and old wives' tales put together. I refer to those doom-sounding words, "The Change of Life."

No wonder we dread this time when it is saddled with such a description. No wonder some of us think, when we have our first menopausal symptom, that the end is at hand.

For of all the stupid phrases ever invented, this is about the most stupid. And of all the misnomers, this takes the prize. Certainly it is a change. But the phrase *the change* makes it sound like the only change. And *change of life* makes it sound as if your whole life is to be different, which is far from the case.

This change is no more the change of your whole life than all the other changes which have gone before and will come after. For living is constant change; that is its essence. One of the best definitions of living is by George Lewes: "A living thing is something that is always changing, yet always remaining essentially the same."

Mull over those words, and you'll see what they mean: always changing, but remaining essentially the same. They mean that you are different from a stone or a rock; you're akin to a flower or a tree which changes but remains essentially the same.

The horse chestnut tree outside your window has a blight one year, bears gloriously the next, but you know it's the same tree. The geranium on your windowsill has only one sickly flower now, soon it will be all abloom, but you recognize it to be the same geranium. It's the same with you. You have been changing ever since the moment you were conceived, and will continue to change until you make your exit speech.

Think back with me a moment and see if this isn't so.

Probably the greatest change that ever occurred to you happened when you were born—delivered alive and kicking out of the womb. What a change that was! In a few brief minutes you slipped from an untroubled world inside your mother to a workaday world outside. From snug warmth where you lay cozily and sopped up nourishment, to a place where you had to labor hard for every bit of milk.

You really were uncomfortable about that change called birth. But just as you got used to it came another—the change from liquid to solid food. Just as you were getting used to mother's milk or formula it was taken away from you. Life snatched away the tender breast, the comforting bottle, put you through the miseries of teething, and made you grapple with a hard cup and spoon.

Then, as you were getting used to *this* change, came still another. Life thrust you from babyhood into childhood with the command, "You are ready for school!" In a relentless moment you were escorted firmly out of your familiar household and deposited in a strange, cold place where an equally strange person called "Teacher" took you in charge. Now you couldn't even do a simple thing like go to the bathroom when you wanted to; you had to wave your hand and wait until you were told.

Yet you got used to this change also, learned to like it in fact, when, with equal suddenness, you were thrust from childhood into adolescence. Adolescence was a terrible change at first. Oh, the problems of that first menstrual period and those newly budding breasts. The emotional turmoil that stabbed sharp as any knife. The ups and downs and strange sensations—surely as strange as any during the menopause. Who remembers adolescence as a time of pure bliss? Only those poets who have forgotten what it is like to be young.

Then the change from adolescence to young womanhood. How one moment you stood proud on a platform at school graduation, a shining diploma in your hand; yet the next moment were cringing to prospective employers vying for that first job. Talk of drastic upheavals and new sensations! It's only because you've been comparatively placid for so long that you've forgotten the upheavals of those days.

And so the story goes. . . .

The great emotional change the first time you made love. The startling change when your first baby arrived, and you realized in a moment of panic that you could no longer remain the irresponsible child of your mother, but must become the responsible mother of your child.

Think back on all these or changes like them—things you have weathered, things you have learned to take in your stride—and you will see how downright wicked it was to have called this particular change, which is merely one among others, THE change of life.

True, you are older now. True, this one looms large and so seems harder to face. But then, as William Carlos Williams says, "Terror enlarges any object, as does joy. 'The whole forest seemed to open,' said the hunter of his first tiger. 'I don't know what its exact size may have been, but to me it seemed thirty feet high.' "

No, it isn't the menopause which is frightening you half so much as the terror surrounding it. It really looks thirty feet high. And most of the terror comes from that phrase I hate even to go on mentioning—"The change of life."

Most Germans don't use that phrase. They use a kinder one: *Die wechseljahre.*

Most French people don't use it. They use an even kinder one: *Le retour a l'age,* or "The return to the age." They imply by this a return to the age before the time of fertility. A return to some of the carefree days.

So why should you and I use it? Why not use some of those truer phrases like, "Another change," or "The changing years?"

I suggest you practice those right now. Say: "I'm going through another change." Or: "I'm going through the changing years." You'll be surprised how much this simple word substitution will do for your frame of mind.

Let's start now with the first clue to the puzzle and see why it is just another change.

3

The Mystery of Your Glands

If your grandmother had taken a stroll down Main Street some fifty odd years ago and met her friend Susan, and Susan had asked, "How are you feeling today?" your grandmother may have replied: "Not so well. I haven't been myself lately. Must be my liver, I guess. Or maybe my heart."

But if you were to take the same stroll today, and the same question was put, you might have a different explanation. Instead of blaming your heart or liver, you might be very modern and blame your hormones.

For hormone knowledge is new. So new it goes back only to the late nineteenth century, and to a remarkable Frenchman named Brown-Séquard.

BROWN-SÉQUARD AND HIS DOG ESSENCE

On a warm June evening in Paris, in the year 1889, a distinguished old gentleman named Charles Édouard Brown-Séquard made a startling announcement to some fellow scientists.

"Messieurs," he said, "all my life, as you know, I have been a hard worker. But lately my strength, which was at one time great, has considerably diminished. Up until two weeks ago I was so weak I had to sit down instead of stand in the laboratory. And when I got home, all I could do was partake of a meager supper and go straight to bed."

But then, he went on, this amazing thing happened: He had started giving himself a series of injections; he had removed the testicles from some young and vigorous dogs, boiled these down into a concentrate, and injected this concentrate into himself.

"Behold the results," he continued. "Miracle of miracles, and wonder of wonders. After only a few injections I can work for hours. I stand up in the laboratory instead of sitting down. And when I get home, I eat a hearty supper and return once more to my work."

His colleagues scoffed at first, but Brown-Séquard continued his experiments, and when he reported the same results a few weeks later they burst into applause.

It was as if a bomb had exploded in that quiet Paris room. Newspapers blazoned his discovery in huge type on their front pages. Learned societies discussed it. It looked as if the Fountain of Youth had been found at last.

For come to think of it, mused the scientists, they should have suspected one answer to strength might lie in the testicles. *Of course* these sex glands had more than mere "sex" functions. *Certainly* they were connected with general health.

Take eunuchs, for example. Deprived of his testicles, a eunuch lost far more than the power to reproduce. The shape of his body was altered. His muscular strength was lessened. His nervous tone was lowered. He tired more easily, became irritable and moody. Surely no one could sneak a glance into a harem and confuse the deprived eunuch with the intact Sultan, even though both at the moment happened to be lounging in identical fancy pajamas and fez.

Then there were farm animals. Almost everybody knew how the fierce bull after alteration became the docile ox. How the cock or rooster, caponized to make his meat more tender, became far less "cocky." How the altered tomcat slept long by the fire instead of continuing to roam.

Yes, surely sex was in some way connected with vigor and strength. Take the sex glands *out* of a body and it became changed—of that there was no doubt. But put sex glands back *in?* In spite of Brown-Séquard, the results of doing this were still far from clear.

So, careful, quiet scientists kept working away at the problem in laboratories. For at least thirty years they worked, until their persistence paid off. While they found nothing even faintly resembling an elixir people could gulp to keep them eternally young, they did find medicines of great help for certain times in our lives. Help for women especially, and very especially for the changing years. In the 1920s these medicines, called hormones, were dramatically announced.

As one doctor put it: "In the 1920s the whole story of the hormones burst like a meteor on the medical profession. . . . The whole amazing concept of the influence of the hormones on a woman's economy astonished the medical world."

There could no longer be any doubt about it. The sex glands have an almost magical influence on many aspects of our lives. Once you know this influence, the menopause can no longer be the mystery to you it was to your grandmother.

THE FOUR MAGICAL GLANDS

The sex glands, however, are only part of the story. The quiet scientists in the laboratories found many others. For our purpose four are the most important. But these four provide one of the main clues to why you may get upset and tired during your changing years, and why, once this time is over, you will be yourself again.

Perhaps the easiest way to start to understand these main glands is to picture yourself in a railway train being carried speedily from New York to Chicago. You are warm. You are comfortable. You know you're being safely carried along.

If you give any thought as to why you are safe, you think only about the car in which you are seated. The car is strong and secure. Maybe once in a while you give a thought to the motorman running the train from his cab up front—certainly the motorman's more important than the car. But there you stop. You forget the great system of distant power stations and signals that are blinking their red and green lights—the signals that are really keeping you on the track.

Well, compare the railway cars to the parts of your body you are usually pretty much aware of—such as your heart, stomach, or lungs. Compare the motorman to your brain that "runs" these parts. And compare the power stations, those distant places that supply the spark that in turn runs the whole outfit—compare these to the tiny, remote power plants in your body, your endocrine glands.

The key to the puzzle of the menopause lies in four of the endocrine glands—the pituitary or master gland, the thyroid, adrenal, and the ovaries. First let's look at your thyroid, or energy gland.

Your Thyroid or Energy Gland

Buttonhole a group of people and ask them where their energy comes from. Nine chances out of ten you'll get the answer, "Why, from the food I eat."

Well, food is not quite the answer. Food is important, surely. But it's only an energy ingredient, like oil in a furnace or flour in a cake. The spark that sets the oil burning is your thyroid gland.

A fast-burning thyroid, powered by the pituitary, explains a dynamic Sammy Davis, the kind of man who, in his fifties, still sings with vim and dances like a puppet on strings. Or a Toscanini, who at eighty could conduct a ten-hour symphony rehearsal, then bound up the stairs when he got home, calling out to his wife to get ready to join him in a walk. Or a Bernard Shaw who in his nineties remarked to an overenthusiastic visitor: "Get along with you. I'm already three years behind in my work as it is!"

On the other hand, people born with a slow-burning thyroid act the opposite way. They are dull, lethargic. Many "backward" children simply need to take a little extra thyroid extract. Indeed, doctors say there is nothing more exciting in the whole realm of medicine than to see a youngster who was dismissed as dull-witted come alive after treatment with thyroid extract.

The thyroid, then, is a great energy gland—a tiny furnace that makes your life fires burn bright. It sparks your body, it sparks your mind. It's so powerful that there are never more than about three and a half grains of pure thyroid hormone (thyroxine) circulating within your body at a time. Yet a variation in that three and a half grains can make all the difference between being half asleep and vibrantly alive.

What is more, thyroxine keeps circulating through your bloodstream in a steady rhythm as a rule. It is only at certain times of stress, such as the menopause, that it may lose that steady rhythm. How and why this happens we'll soon see.

Your Sex Glands or Stimulating Glands

The next set of glands which may act up during the menopause are your sex or stimulating glands, your ovaries.

Why do we call your ovaries your stimulating glands? You probably always have thought of them mainly as reproductive glands, but they are far more than that. They also stimulate your entire body. Like your thyroid, they supply you with energy that fires your life spark.

From the moment you are born until the moment you die, sex power is also energy power, keeping your heart pumping quietly, your brain thinking clearly, and your blood flowing evenly along its course.

So your ovaries have a double purpose. They are reproductive glands, but also energy glands. To sum up their double job, we call them your stimulating glands.

Your Adrenal or Emergency Glands

If your sex glands are amazing, your adrenals are even more so. These are two-in-one glands, having a core or center, and a rim. The adrenals supply the day-to-day energy (by means of a secretion of cortisol) that regulates carbohydrate, fat, and protein metabolism. The core supplies you with still another kind of energy

—emergency energy. The core of the adrenals produces chemicals that come out in little squirts whenever an extra amount of energy is needed, and in big squirts when real emergencies arise. Think of them this way:

If you were just a plowhorse, your thyroid and sex glands might be enough to take care of your energy needs. But you are more than a plowhorse; you are also a racehorse; life consists of far more than jogging along. Almost everyday there are moments when a special kind of energy is called for. Moments of hunger or cold. Of sudden fatigue or stress. Of danger, illness, or fear. Moments when you must gather from somewhere the strength to fight or to run like the wind to preserve your life.

So the wise organism that is your body has prepared you for such things too. Like a woman who has food in the refrigerator for tonight's dinner, but also has reserves in the freezer for unexpected guests, nature has prepared you to meet emergencies as well. And your emergency department lies within your adrenal glands.

Let a hunter be pursued by a wild beast and run for it. It's his adrenals that give him the power to leap over brooks far too wide for him to leap ordinarily, to run both faster and longer without feeling fatigue.

Let an army captain hear that the enemy, superior in numbers, is nearer than he suspected and order his exhausted men on. It's the adrenals that call out from hidden places in the soldiers' bodies extra supplies of blood sugar and enable them to march some more.

Or let your child be taken ill and face a crisis. It's your adrenals that give you the endurance to stand vigil without sleep or food by his bedside, stand twenty-four hours, thirty-six hours, forty-eight hours if need be, though ordinarily you would have dropped in your tracks.

Even when you are confronted with an excess of joy that makes your heart beat so loud you can hear it, your pulse beat so loud you can feel it, it's your adrenals that have caused this pleasure reaction. In fact, under any kind of intense emotional need or excitement, it's your adrenals that provide the rush of energy.

It was Dr. Walter Cannon, Harvard professor and researcher extraordinary, who first told the world about the adrenals. Until Cannon began the work which culminated in his great book *Bodily Changes in Pain, Hunger, Fear and Rage,* centuries of research had turned up only these few unrelated facts:

One: Your adrenals, located above your kidneys and hardly larger than a quarter of a dollar, still have the richest blood supply of any organ of the body; seven and a half times their own weight in blood passes through them every minute—even more than through the heart or brain.

Two: When adrenal extract is injected into a person his heart pumps faster and his blood circulates more speedily (though his digestion stops cold and a complete bowel evacuation often occurs).

Three: The adrenal glands are the only glands which are absolutely necessary for a body to function. When the adrenals are removed from an experimental animal it almost immediately curls up and dies.

Cannon put these known facts together and did a lot of thinking. What, he asked, could at the same time make the heart beat faster, the blood race quicker, digestion stop, and the bowels unload? Nothing but danger. An emergency. A need to make a quick change. Confronted with these, all the body's vital activities are speeded up to prepare for fight or flight. The bowels unload to lighten the body, while digestion, which is a luxury, can wait.

Tiny organs like the adrenals need their rich blood supply so that they can be geared for fast action. An animal deprived of its adrenals will die because it can no longer cope with dangers or emergencies. Deprived of its adrenals it is helpless—at the mercy of every wind that blows.

Later researchers confirmed Cannon's work. They proved that during any kind of stress it's your adrenals that come to your rescue and pour out their hormones in large spurts. They help you during the changes your body faces during severe illness. They help you during the stress of pregnancy. They help you during daily stresses such as going from extreme heat to extreme cold. And during the stress called the menopause? As you'll see, they come to your rescue once more.

Your Pituitary or Chief Gland

There's an old army saying: "If it's the bugler's job to wake up the camp each morning, whose job is it to wake up the bugler?"

We come now to a gland that is even more remarkable, if possible, than the adrenals. It's your pituitary or master gland, the one that in a sense wakes up the bugler. In fact, it wakes up all the buglers—your thyroid gland, ovaries, adrenals, and the other endocrine glands down the line. And as befitting a chief or master, your pituitary lies in your skull just under the base of your brain.

Take your ovaries. You were born with fully formed ovaries, but until puberty they were small, half asleep. If your pituitary had not secreted the substances that awakened your ovaries at the proper moment, they may have stayed asleep. But between the ages of eleven and fourteen, as a rule, your pituitary woke them up and the great change called adolescence began.

Your pituitary also awakens and directs your thyroid. To prove this, the famous brain surgeon, Dr. Harvey Cushing, managed by a delicate operation to remove part of a dog's pituitary gland. His thyroid shriveled as a result; he became lazy, languid, and fat; his speed of living slowed to a walk. Still his thyroid itself had not been touched—only the pituitary gland which gave the thyroid its spark.

Then other scientists did Cushing's experiment backward, and found that if a thyroid gland was removed the pituitary was affected. If a sex gland was removed, the chief gland was affected again.

Thus they found that the glands are not independent. Instead, they are members of a network.

How does this network work? The endocrine glands are not like some of the other gland systems, such as the sweat glands, which secrete the substances used in the vicinity of the gland. The endocrine glands are located far from the parts of the body they affect—the thyroid is in the neck, the ovaries of women are in the abdomen, the adrenals right above the kidneys, and the pituitary just under the base of the brain. Since they are far apart, how do they affect each other, as well as your digestion and breathing, and the beating of your heart?

The Mystery is Solved

The mystery was solved when it was discovered that the glands influence each other and the rest of the body by means of a substance called a *hormone.*

Hormone is a word you've been seeing around quite a bit lately. You've seen it on packages of hormone creams; on bottles of hormone medicine. It comes from the Greek word hormōn, meaning "I arouse" or "I set in action." Hormones thus are substances secreted by the glands which send chemical messages to other glands and set them in action.

Just as a railroad uses radio signals to send out messages from its central power station to set various trains in motion, so do your glands use chemical messages poured into your bloodstream. It is your bloodstream that acts as a radio system to carry these messages around.

Day in and day out these hormone messages travel through your bloodstream. They go back and forth from one gland to another. They also go from your glands to your heart, stomach, nerves, and brain.

THE GAME OF SEESAW

But here's something equally interesting: your glands not only *arouse* each other or set each other in motion, they also *calm down* or *stop* each other at certain times.

It works this way: Your chief gland, the pituitary, sends out a chemical message—say to your ovaries at ovulation time—a message telling them to get busy and release an egg. Your ovaries respond by pouring out hormones. But when they have poured out enough hormones to discharge an egg, your ovaries send back a message saying, "Stop!"

At another time, your pituitary sends a message to your thyroid, calling for an energy burst because it's summertime and you have a long day of gardening ahead. Then, when your thyroid has produced so much energy that it is in danger of getting overtired, it calms down your pituitary by sending back a message to halt production.

It all works out something like an old-fashioned balance-scale. Your pituitary is on one end of the scale and a gland on the other. When the pituitary end is up, the other goes down. When another gland is up, the pituitary goes down.

Also, as in any scale the saw never quite reaches a state of balance. There is a constant movement toward balance, but never a perfect achievement of it.

This is probably the most important single thing to remember to fully understand the menopause: *Throughout your entire life your glands are always moving toward balance but never quite achieving it. They never come entirely to rest.*

Yet strangely enough you're seldom aware of all this movement. It goes on quietly within you as a rule. Certain times, however, are exceptions. Then the scale swings up and down harder than usual and you notice it—sometimes with a vengeance.

One of these noticing times can be the menopause.

A rabbi was asked to give the essence of religion while standing on one foot. He replied: "The essence of religion is to love thy neighbor as thyself."

If anyone were to ask you to give the essence of the menopause while standing on one foot, you could reply: "The menopause is a time when my gland scale swings up and down harder than usual, and I notice it as a result."

The Scale Calms Down Again

Yet strangest of all, just as the scale swings up and down more than usual during the menopause, it comes back to its comparatively calm state after your menopause is over.

How does this return come about? Ah, that's the "plot" of this book! And frankly, as in a mystery story, I'm not ready to tell it yet. But here's a hint: The scale calms down after the menopause by a change of partners.

At different stages in your life your pituitary seems to have a more-or-less favorite partner that balances it.

During childhood, when your ovaries were not yet mature, this favorite partner was your adrenal glands.

When menstruation arrived, your ovaries became its favorite partner instead.

But now that the menopause is arriving and your ovaries are withdrawing, your chief gland must find a new partner.

How does it do this? Read on.

4

Menstruation: A Tide Rises and Falls

No one forgets her first menstrual period. We remember it for two reasons: It is surrounded by mystery. It has to do with blood.

To most of us, the sight of blood is horrifying because it spells trouble. If we are cut or hit hard, blood flows. If we are severely wounded, blood flows once more. And blood, we have been told, is the precious life substance. To lose even a small quantity can be dangerous. To lose a lot can bring on hemorrhage or death.

Now suddenly we lose a lot of blood, and lose it for mysterious reasons. We haven't been cut or hit; we haven't been wounded. Where does this particular blood come from? Consequently we are frightened and baffled at the same time.

More, we lose this baffling blood from a place that up to now has been strange and forbidden; lose it in a way over which we have no control. If we have not been prepared for the experience, we may panic. Has the genital play we may have indulged in for a while anything to do with it? Is the uncontrolled flow something for which we will be punished, as we may have been punished as a child for wetting our pants? Or worse, is it evidence of some mysterious disease?

Havelock Ellis tells of a suicide attempt after a first menstruation. In his classic *Studies in the Psychology of Sex,* he tells this story:

"A few years ago a case was reported in the French newspapers of a young girl of 15, who threw herself into the Seine at Saint-Ouen. She was rescued and on being brought before the police commissioner said that she had been attacked by an 'unknown disease.' Discreet inquiry revealed that the mysterious malady was one common to all women and the girl was restored to her insufficiently punished parents."

Of course, few girls react in a way as extreme as attempted suicide. But far more girls reach puberty without knowledge of the subject than most people realize, and statistics show that only a small percentage of girls really understand menstruation before it happens to them, even in these modern days.

NOT LISTENING

This lack of knowledge, however, is not always as much the parents' fault as Havelock Ellis implies. Some mothers honestly do try to tell their daughters about menstruation before it happens. But Dr. Helene Deutsch makes the point that many girls deny they have been told anything for the simple reason they were not listening. Memory is always selective, so no matter how many questions girls may have asked on this or other subjects relating to sex, they usually have not been listening to the answers if these answers were unpleasant, especially if they came from someone as close as a mother. They therefore often forget what they have learned, and have to learn it all over again later when the matter has become more urgent.

HIDDEN HOSTILITY

Or we may deny advance knowledge because of hidden hostility to our mothers, since some mothers say incorrect or insensitive things, usually as a result of their own discomfort in explaining menstruation to their daughters.

There is, for instance, Eleanor, whose mother used menstruation for teasing. Eleanor as a child was very thin. When other women were present, her mother would often remark on this thinness, then giggle and hint that "someday something would happen to fill her out." But she refused to tell Eleanor what this something was, merely tittering "You'll see!" as if the matter were some private grown-up joke.

Her first menstruation came by chance to Eleanor the day after she had taken a ride on a roller coaster. She became petrified at the unexpected blood and figured the ride had something to do with it. Maybe it had injured her somehow; or maybe now she would need an operation and the "filling out" would come as a result. Nor did it help when her mother dismissed the matter curtly: "This is what I was expecting. Now forget about it, except to remember it will come back next month." How could she forget, especially when it didn't come back the next month, or the next? Menstruation is so intimately connected with the nervous system that fear can easily suppress it. In Eleanor's case, she was so frightened she didn't have a period again for a year.

Dr. A. E. Rackoff of the Jefferson Medical School points out that it is quite common not to menstruate regularly for months or even years after the start of the flow—to be irregular in frequency, amount, and length of days, since the pituitary and ovaries are not yet working in a well-regulated partnership. But in this case the natural tendency was greatly heightened by fear.

Then Josephine's mother used menstruation as a punishment. Josephine had just gone through the normal tomboy stage and when her first period arrived her mother announced: "That's what you get for climbing trees. Now you're splitting up the middle as a result." I don't have to say what a fearful thought "splitting up the middle" is. It was enough to stop Josephine too for a year.

On the day of Jennie's first period, her mother gave her daughter a hard slap across her face. Jennie also thought the slap was a punishment, if not for climbing trees, then for doing the "dirty thing" of uncontrollably menstruating. Actually, the slap was done in accordance with an old notion you had to slap a newly menstruating girl to keep the color in her face, since otherwise she would lose her color because "all her blood was running out the other end."

Of course, few mothers behave in these extreme ways. Some avoid the matter because it seems such a touchy subject they just can't bring themselves to discuss it. So either they postpone it until the last minute or, if they do bring it up, they run through it like a steamroller as something to be gotten over fast. And other mothers, knowing that many schools have sex education courses as required parts of the curriculum, just leave it up to the schools, whose teachers sometimes also do a hurried, embarrassed job.

Menstrual Blood as Poisonous

One reason mothers and teachers sometimes are so embarrassed is that they find it hard to get over old beliefs imbibed from *their* mothers—beliefs like those that preach menstruating women are "poisonous" or "unclean."

The belief that they are poisonous is very old. Some cultures believed they were so poisonous that menstruating women were segregated in special menstrual huts where they were served special foods from special pots, after which the pots were destroyed for fear they might be used again and contaminate the entire tribe. (Indeed, some cultures still segregate menstruating women.) Other cultures slung up newly menstruating girls in dark huts in hammocks, stung them with nettles, or made them wear special bonnets that hung down over their faces to protect men from their "evil eyes." And the Roman writer Pliny was quoted for centuries after he declared that if a menstruating woman entered the door of a winery, the wine would turn sour; if she stirred milk, it would curdle; if she sewed, the thread would knot; if she touched flowers, the flowers would die.

England's Mary Chadwick thinks things like the segregation in dark huts, and the stinging with nettles, were forms of initiation rites, testing a girl's fitness to enter womanhood as many societies test boys; while the slinging up in the dark in hammocks is symbolic of being halfway between heaven and earth, or between death and rebirth, to symbolize the fact a girl is now dying as a child and being reborn into a new life.

As to blaming women for wine that turned sour, or grain that withered, primitive people don't take chances with their precious possessions. By sheer chance a woman who is menstruating may have entered a winery the day a batch of wine was ready to go bad, walked across a field just before a drought that caused the grain to wither. And since people like dramatic stories, they blew up these happenings into a Big Deal.

Menstrual Blood as Good

Yet not all the stories have to do with blame. Some cultures have believed the blood of menstruating women to be powerful and good. A medieval tale held that if a warrior's sword were whetted with it, his sword would become doubly keen. An Italian belief had it that if an unfertile woman borrowed a sanitary napkin from a fertile woman, she would become blessed with children. Still other people gave a menstruating woman the awesome power of foretelling the future, or raising up storms against an enemy at sea.

Biblical Beliefs

The tales of a menstruating woman's danger, however, have outweighed the tales of her power, since they have been unhappily reinforced by the Bible. It was the Bible that used the word "unclean" to describe menstruating women, and many biblical scholars think this was a most unfortunate term since the same word was used to describe lepers.

But by unclean the Bible meant "ritually unclean." When a so-called "issue of blood" was coming forth from her body, an orthodox Jewish woman could not join in any sacred ritual, or touch any hallowed thing. She had to remain separate and apart until she had gone through a purification bath, the mikvah, before she could rejoin the group. And today in Israel, orthodox men also have to take similar baths after a nocturnal emission, which is called "nocturnal pollution." This is another unfortunate choice of words since, like menstruation, it is hardly something within a man's control.

But semen, like blood, has also been considered both good and bad. Good because it could bring about conception; bad because it could spread venereal disease. The Israeli bath is to "wash the man clean." And since these baths are communal baths, the men and women who take them splash around, gossip, and in general have a fine time.

So the beliefs about menstruation swing from good to bad, while the hormone tides, in their rise and fall, bring things both good and bad as well.

OTHER GOOD AND BAD RESULTS

One good result of the hormone rise is what happens in pregnancy.

During pregnancy estrogen literally floods the body; it increases to almost twenty times the normal amount. As a result, a woman may feel and look radiant. Also, the level of the hormone progesterone goes way up. Since progesterone is in some ways a quieting hormone it can make a woman placid and turn her still further inward as if listening to an inner clock. As Eva put it, "When I'm pregnant I feel as if I'm on the deck of a boat that is smoothly sailing along. I don't have to do anything, but I reach port just the same."

MORE GOOD INTERPRETATIONS

Then there's the modern discovery that many things the body throws off are not poisonous at all.

Some are the result of an infection, and so doctors handle them with great care. But menstrual blood is a natural, noninfectious product, so they handle it freely. Indeed, many doctors prefer to give women gynecological exams during their periods because the uterus and cervix are more open. They insert IUDs at that time for the same reason.

Also, doctors have known for a long time that urine is not poisonous either. Before there were special tests for diabetes, they used to taste a bit of the patient's urine to see if it tasted sweet. If it did, it turned out to be quite an accurate way of diagnosing the disease.

In fact, with rare exceptions, practically nothing thrown off by the body is toxic or poisonous. And this is true for both women and men.

The Truth About Menstruation

We don't yet know everything about menstruation. But we do know a great deal.

We know for instance that menstruation is not being "unwell" or "the curse" anymore than being tired and hungry is being "unwell" or "a curse." True, many women feel somewhat low at the time, but that's not the same thing as being unwell or ill.

We know too that, since it is not "bad blood" you are not automatically hurt if you never menstruate, or menstruate seldom. (I have a friend who has periods every three months; another friend mysteriously stopped for seven years, then for no apparent reason started up again. Aside from the fact she couldn't conceive during this time, she suffered no harm.) And you are certainly not hurt when you stop altogether, as after the menopause. You certainly can no longer conceive, but there's no automatic harm or loss.

We know too that a menstrual cycle can vary from twenty-one to forty-five days and still be normal. The twenty-eight-day cycle is merely a statistical average. It is also normal for the same woman to have a period, say, twenty-seven days after her last one, then have to wait thirty-two days before the next. All kinds of things can affect the cycle, for instance, a change of climate. Airline attendants, who leave New Orleans in the morning and land in the Andes at night, can have their cycles drastically affected because of changes in altitude. Women who fear pregnancy can have their cycles affected by anxiety. Many factors can be at play.

As Dr. S. Leon Israel puts it: "The absolutely regular menstrual cycle is so rare as to be either a myth or a medical curiosity." Women who desire a regular cycle can now get it by taking the birth-control pill under a doctor's guidance. Usually estrogen alone is taken for a certain number of days, then estrogen combined with progesterone. When the medication is stopped, menstruation, in this instance called "withdrawal bleeding," takes place.

Let us compare the menstrual month to a three-act drama, with the pituitary and ovarian glands as the chief actors. We will see that within this three-act drama, there is a hidden moment which is the high point of the play, as well as tides that rise and fall.

THE THREE-ACT DRAMA OF MENSTRUATION

The drama opens at puberty with an overture or prologue, as most plays do. This is the sending out by your ovaries of a large quantity of sex hormones known as the *estrogens*. Under the stimulus of your chief gland, which in turn is controlled by the hypothalamus, a first full tide is sent out. As it rushes out, the menstrual play is ready to begin, the pituitary and ovaries working together in a stop and go arrangement.

Estrogen is a Greek word. It comes from *estros* meaning "desire" or "heat"; and *gennao* meaning "to produce." Estrogen is thus "the hormone which produces heat or desire," i.e., sexual desire *in* a woman, and desire *for* her on the part of a man. Without its kindly influence one might never attract, or be attracted to, a mate.

Some estrogen has been released by your ovaries since infancy, and there was enough to be counted from about the age of four. Around the age of seven the amount took a sharp upswing, and by the age of eight there was usually enough to color the tiny nipples of your breast a deeper pink. But it was not until later that the tide rose really high—high enough to cause your first menstrual period to appear.

This first high tide, moreover, brought with it other blessings as well. It beautified and energized your entire body. Rounded your figure. Softened your skin. Energized your mind and emotions, too. Do you remember the great burst of intellectual curiosity that characterized your adolescence? The possible fervor for poetry, religion, or music? You can largely thank that great tide of estrogen for these.

Curiously, though, this first tide, though it brings menstruation, may not also bring fertility. We are apt to think that as soon as we menstruate we are ready to conceive. That is not always the case. In fact, in countries like India where it is the custom for men to take very young girls as brides, fewer babies arrive than one might expect. This is because girls are not fertile as a rule until around the age of fifteen, though younger girls who trust this to be so, and have sex without using birth control, may find themselves unpleasantly surprised, especially since they are also thrown off by the fact that menstruation is so often irregular during the first few years. But after age fifteen menstrual periods usually come steadily month after month, your pituitary joining with your ovaries to bring this about.

And with their regular arrival, the curtain rises on the Menstrual Month, a drama in which waves rise and fall.

Act I: The First Wave Rises and Falls

We will assume a standard menstrual month of twenty-eight days, of which the first day of the flow is called Day One. And since the flow lasts for four days on the average, the day after it stops becomes Day Five. Day Five is when the drama actually begins, for it is then that a hormone wave begins to rise. On Day Five your pituitary sends a message to your ovaries telling them to "go"—that is to pour out estrogen; it is this estrogen that, as its level rises, causes the first up wave.

As the wave rises, your ovaries begin to ripen an ovum or

egg. On Days Five through Fourteen the ripening goes on while the wave rises still more.

On or about Day Fourteen comes the climax. The estrogen wave reaches its highest peak; an egg ripens and is released from the ovary. The moment of release is called ovulation. If there were a musical accompaniment to the drama, on Ovulation Day you would hear a cymbal crash.

Curiously, on Ovulation Day your body temperature goes down sharply, then goes up about half a degree. Most of us run a daily temperature, barring illness, of 98.6° F. On Ovulation Day it goes up to around 99.2° F. So one way you can determine whether you are ovulating is to take a daily temperature reading before breakfast. If there is an upward jump around Day Fourteen of .04 to .08 of a degree, you know one of your ovaries has released an egg.

Another way to tell if you've ovulated, one which doctors often use, is to look for changes in the consistency of your cervical mucus. Doctors put a drop of this mucus on a glass slide and look at it through a microscope. On Ovulation Day the appearance of the mucus changes to a fern-like pattern, making ovulation a dramatic moment indeed.

INTERMISSION TIME

With ovulation completed, the first act of the menstrual drama is over. As in most plays, there is an intermission time, during which your ovaries send a "stop" hormone message to your pituitary, so that as a result it takes a brief rest.

Act II: Another Wave
Rises and Falls

Intermission over, the egg that burst forth on Ovulation Day begins to travel down into one of your Fallopian tubes. There it rests for a while, waiting to meet up with a sperm.

Soon after its rest, your pituitary gets busy again. It now prods your ovaries into a new spurt of activity, a spurt that is in some ways greater than before. For until now your ovaries have produced only one hormone, estrogen, the hormone which ripened the egg. But since this egg may become fertilized and start a baby, your ovaries have to work doubly hard to prepare for this possibility. They have to continue to make estrogen as before, but they must also make a second hormone which will nourish the egg if it does become fertilized. This second hormone is called *progesterone,* from *gest* meaning *birth or gestation,* and *pro* meaning *in favor of.* Progesterone can thus be called the in-favor-of birth hormone, since its job here is to thicken and make ready with rich blood the lining of your uterus—make as it were a "nest" for the fertilized egg so it can rest and grow there.

Under the guidance of your pituitary, then, Act II finds your ovaries rising in a double wave, for they are making both progesterone and estrogen. The purpose of the estrogen is to continue to energize your whole body; progesterone to enrich and make ready the nest-lining of your uterus.

So up, up, up during Act II your pituitary and ovaries work together to make that double wave, until another message is sent back to your pituitary to stop and briefly rest.

Act III: The Double Wave
Rises and Falls

As the last days of the month approach, or around Days Twenty-two and Twenty-four, your pituitary starts up once more. As a result the double wave reaches its peak. If the egg which burst forth on Ovulation Day has been fertilized, well and good; your uterus is ready to receive it. If not, well and good again. The un-fertilized egg will crumble and slip out through your vagina, and next month your pituitary and ovary will patiently repeat the whole drama of the menstrual month so far.

But there is more to come. For nature is not only patient, she is generous. She is the kind of housekeeper who wouldn't dream of serving leftovers for food. So just as she discards an egg that hasn't been fertilized, she discards an unused uterine lining too.

This is what menstruation really is—the discharge of a few tablespoons of blood from the unused uterine lining. Yes it's only a few—though it's mixed with so many enzymes and other material it looks like more. And according to Dr. George Friedman, you lose so little iron in these few tablespoons you don't need iron supplements unless your flow happens to be unusually heavy, and when that happens, get a small amount of the cheapest iron you can find. For remember, iron is constipating, and if you tend to have cramps, constipation will only make them worse.

THE THREE-ACT DRAMA CAUSES EMOTIONAL CHANGES TOO

The three-act drama of menstruation also causes emotional changes throughout the month.

These emotional changes have until now been almost as mysterious as the physical changes. Why does a woman sometimes feel heavy and irritable a few days before her menstrual flow—so irritable that even her best friends notice it—not to mention her husband?

Why does she feel "low" during the flow itself, either during the entire time or just the first day? And why does she bounce back and feel herself again after the flow is over?

As one woman put it: "Why do I hate my job, hate my boss, hate my home, hate everything before or during menstruation, yet love them all again once it is through? And why each month do I forget all about last month, and go through the same cycle of emotions again?"

Before we can answer these questions, let's take a quick look once more at the three main menstrual acts, remembering that sex hormones are also stimulating hormones to the entire body.

Act I includes Days Five through Fourteen. This is egg-ripening time, when a big wave of estrogen is flooding you with stimulating hormones, rising to a peak around Day Fourteen. On or about Day Fourteen (Ovulation Day) the crest of the first wave is reached. This is followed by a short dip or rest.

Act II includes Days Fourteen to Twenty-eight. Now there is a double hormone wave, for this is preparing-of-the-uterus time, when progesterone is added to estrogen. Again there is a peak around Day Twenty-four. But after this peak, instead of taking merely a short dip, the waves dip down sharply. During Days Twenty-four to Twenty-eight they dip down so sharply they sink to the low point of the month.

Act III, or the menstrual period itself, is the trough of the wave. The fall has been so deep it is now really "low tide." These hormone peaks and valleys are the clues to your feeling ups and downs.

During menstruation (on Days One to Five), when your hormone production is low, you may feel low and miserable and full of the blues.

When menstruation is over and the wave shoots up again, you feel fine—ready to lick the world.

As the wave climbs steadily higher and higher toward Ovulation Day, you feel better and better.

On or about Ovulation Day you feel at your peak.

Then comes a short feeling dip as the wave slightly drops, followed by another high feeling point, possibly the highest of all, around Day Twenty-four. For both estrogen and progesterone are at the summit to stimulate you now. You are really "rarin' to go."

But there's a paradox to Day Twenty-four. Not all women feel well. On the contrary, some women can't tolerate quite so much hormone at once. For these the seesaw has swung so high they feel overstimulated or tense. Then the office worker complains: "My head aches like mad." The housewife says: "My breasts are so swollen and uncomfortable they feel twice their size." The high-school girl declares: "I got on the scale yesterday and I've gained three whole pounds!"

Yet all this results merely from what doctors call "premenstrual tension" or water retention caused by too much hormone. Within the next few days, when the excess goes, the weight will miraculously disappear, the headache will vanish, the breasts subside.

The wave will dip down from high to low, bringing with it menstruation. Soon everything will be fine again as a new cycle begins.

And so the monthly pendulum swings in all women, back and forth, back and forth, back and forth once more. There is a striving toward balance but never quite an achievement of balance. The scale never comes completely to rest.

The pendulum swings for men, too, but not so vigorously or noticeably. Men also have their cycles of ups and downs. But women feel theirs more—of that there is no doubt.

But though women may feel their cycles more than men do, this is not to say that it will affect their performance on a job. There is still a lot of prejudice about hiring women, especially for jobs that involve decision-making, with management using the excuse that, because of their swings, "women are apt to be undependable during certain days of the month." Nonsense. They are no more undependable than men. Men, for instance, drink as a rule much more than women do; as a result there is a tremendous amount of absence on Mondays because of hangovers, when men call in and say they have colds or pneumonia. (The day is often jokingly referred to as "Pneumonia Monday.") And what about John F. Kennedy, whose health swung up and down because of both a bad back and a disease that caused a progressive deterioration of his adrenal glands? Or Thomas Jefferson, who was subject all his life to debilitating migraine headaches? Or Abraham Lincoln, who had spells of terrible depression that caused his pendulum very sharply to swing? Their performance on the job didn't suffer to any noticeable extent. (Management is slowly coming to realize that such things are individual matters.)

Back to Women's Swings

Going back to women's swings, there are large swings in addition to the monthly ones. There is, for instance, the great swing of pregnancy.

We learn here why a limited number of pregnancies are good for a woman, and why many women feel so well and look so radiant during pregnancy when beneficial sex hormones literally *flood* their bodies. To be sure, all change is upsetting at first, especially such a violent change as pregnancy, so during the first few weeks there may be many internal adjustments to make. But after that? Many women positively bloom.

The swing also explains why after delivery there is, for a time, neither menstruation nor ovulation, especially if a woman is nursing a child. Women have whispered to each other for centuries: "Nurse long, my dear, if you do not wish to conceive again soon." This old notion turns out, however, to be only partly true. For while a mother is nursing a baby her pituitary largely switches from stimulating her ovaries to produce eggs, to stimulating her breasts to make the milk-secreting hormone prolactin. And when little or no ovarian hormone is being made, there is usually no ovulation, hence no new conception. But this is not always the case. Drs. Mazer and Goldstein did a study on twelve hundred women and found that fifty-five percent of them did begin to ovulate again while nursing, while only forty-five percent did not. So it boils down to about a fifty-fifty chance that a woman may not conceive while nursing a child.

A woman's hormone swing also explains another riddle: why the so-called "rhythm theory" of contraception seldom works. The rhythm theory, as you may know, is based on the fact that a woman is fertile only during those few days around ovulation time. By calculating carefully when ovulation occurs, she can restrict sex to the non-fertile times. But ovulation, alas, is far from fixed. It takes place on or around Day Fourteen only in women who hold pretty much to the twenty-eight-day cycle. In women with shorter cycles, of, say, twenty-one days, Ovulation Day tends to move forward. That is, the last part of the monthly drama takes two weeks as usual. But the first act is shortened to a week. So that in a woman with a twenty-one-day cycle, if you count Day One as the first day of menstruation, ovulation will occur as early as Day Seven. So you can see why all women can't put faith in Day Fourteen.

And of course if you menstruate irregularly, as during the

menopause, you can't trust Day Fourteen at all, because by now a regular time to count from practically doesn't exist.

THE COW AND THE PLACENTA

And, finally, the hormone swing explains the very curious fact of why a cow eats up the placenta or afterbirth as soon as her calf is born. Why should the cow, ordinarily a vegetarian, gobble up the placenta, which is almost pure meat? The cow eats the placenta because it is bursting with the sex hormones made during her pregnancy. And right after giving birth she is greatly depleted of hormones, all the more so in contrast to the high amount she recently had. Instinctively she devours the rich feast of the placenta, taking back into her own body its bountiful supply.

So we see again and again the evidence of the great symphony constantly being played within a woman's body—a symphony with the music rising and falling as the hormone tides rise and fall. These tides rise and fall in a monthly pattern throughout the fertile years. They rise and fall in a larger pattern throughout the great epochs of life—childhood, adolescence, pregnancy. They rise and fall also during the menopause, as we shall soon see.

MORE MENSTRUAL MYSTERIES

Still more menstrual questions and mysteries exist. The question of cramps. The question of "middle pain." The mystery of the girl who hasn't started to menstruate by the age of sixteen. Let's take them one at a time.

What is the right age to start menstruation? There is no one "right age." Eleven or twelve is average in the United States today, but the normal range goes as low as nine and as high as fifteen. If a girl hasn't started by sixteen, she probably has a faulty pituitary that has not been successful in stimulating her ovaries enough to start the process.

Girls of this kind suffer a good deal, since in addition to not menstruating they usually have undeveloped breasts. And while they can cover up their lack of development by athletic and other achievements, as a rule they are miserable underneath, shy and introverted and feeling they don't "belong." It's a toss-up who is more inwardly anxious—the girl who is ready to menstruate and vaguely fears it, or the girl who hasn't started at the expected time.

Dr. Therese Benedek tells of a patient of hers who had not started at the age of twenty-two. She was nearly six feet tall and still growing, with no breasts, no pubic hair, no evidence of ovarian activity. She suffered greatly, she said, because she "felt like a woman though actually she was just a tall little girl." After hormone-medication plus psychotherapy, she began to spot a little, though her menstrual periods were only token periods. But she was grateful for even this small sign of femininity, especially since her breasts began to develop too.

Now theoretically, since it is a girl's pituitary that is at fault in such cases, the medication should be pituitary hormone. But at the present time a reliable pituitary hormone has not been developed for this purpose. The little available is for research mainly, and extremely expensive. So what is given instead is estrogen and progesterone, given as nearly as possible in imitation of their natural production in the body—that is, estrogen throughout the month, progesterone during the second half, then both hormones withheld until the uterine lining that has been built up is shed.

But this is not true menstruation in the sense that it includes ovulation, so the girl cannot become fertile or conceive. And since the hormones used are replacements for those she lacks, they must be taken indefinitely if even token periods are to result.

The earlier the treatment is started after age sixteen, the more chance there is of good results. Dr. Robert N. Rutherford points out that treatment is often delayed by mothers because they fear the necessary vaginal examination "may destroy their daughter's virginity" or be a "potentially traumatic experience." But he believes the trauma of staying infantile and not achieving periods, even token periods, is far greater than the trauma of an examination sympathetically explained and carefully performed.

Besides, a good doctor can often do such an examination through the rectum instead of the vagina, and learn almost as much.

Inducing Ovulation

Not long ago, two doctors, one a Norwegian and one an Italian, succeeded in inducing ovulation in formerly infertile women with huge injections of the special pituitary hormone that is not generally available. These injections were prohibitive in price, often had to be repeated several times, and so far have caused the birth of an unusually large number of twins, triplets, and quads. But they may become perfected—who knows?

Even when a girl does start to menstruate of her own accord around eleven or twelve, she probably does not ovulate for several years anyway, since the development of fertility is a slow process and takes a longer time than does the establishment of menstruation itself. Dr. Ashley Montagu of Princeton tells of studies done on thousands of women all over the world who were married in their early teens and did not use contraceptives of any kind. Comparatively few of them ovulated or conceived until their twenties.

There are of course exceptions. Everyone knows of teenage mothers. And when teenagers do become mothers, they are usually neither physically nor emotionally ready for the task. Physically they are not ready because too early motherhood may stop them from completing their own growth and development. Emotionally, they are not ready because too early motherhood can be overwhelming. And the younger the girl, the more overwhelming it can be.

This is particularly true if she is not married and has to go through the experience alone. In a Salvation Army home for unmarried mothers in Richmond, Va., I saw older teenagers going about the business of caring for their babies with a certain amount of competence. The younger ones were simply going through the motions; they looked positively dazed.

As if to prove that girls in their teens are not intended to become mothers, nature makes the age of maximum fertility between twenty and thirty.

Women who have been married for some time and have been taking the Pill often stop using it in their thirties and are surprised when they find it difficult to conceive. They immediately blame the contraceptive, thinking it has hurt them in some way. Sometimes the Pill does affect fertility, but more often, it is simply that in their thirties their natural fertility has fallen off. It may therefore take them several months or even years to get pregnant, and in their forties still longer, though it is not impossible until after the menopause, as women with so-called "change of life" babies can testify.

MENSTRUAL PAIN

"Woman-pain has seized my body. Let the gods tear this pain out." This inscription, scratched by some nameless Assyrian woman on a clay tablet three thousand years ago, probably refers to menstrual pain. For what girl or woman has not at some time or other suffered from cramps?

Cramps are irregular, shooting, doubling-up pains in the lower abdomen that come with the first day of the flow, last a short while, and then go away. What causes them? Rather unexpectedly, ovulation. Few girls suffer cramps until they ovulate, which as I said usually doesn't occur until several years after menstruation has begun.

Here's the reason ovulation is the cause. During the first half of the month, as you now know, estrogen alone is made by the ovaries. During the second half, estrogen plus progesterone is made. Estrogen builds up the uterine lining a little. Estrogen plus progesterone builds up the lining a lot. You might say a one-layer cake lining is made by estrogen; a two-layer by estrogen plus. Now the uterus has to expel this lining by squeezing motions. Each time the uterus squeezes, a little lining is thrown off. So cramps are irregular rather than continuous. They accompany the squeezes—a cramp for each squeeze.

The uterus of a girl just beginning to ovulate is quite

inefficient at squeezing. It has not yet had time to build up strong muscles that do the job well. Take a month in which ovulation has occurred, so that a two-layer cake has been made. Add to this a uterus that has not yet become efficient at squeezing. The result may be jerky squeezes that give pain, especially on the first day of the flow when there is a comparatively large amount of lining to be thrown out.

Four Important "Buts"

There are several important "buts" that soften this statement.

First, it is not normal to have a lot of cramps. A study of forty-five hundred girls found that few have enough to incapacitate them.

Second, it is not normal to have *severe* cramps continue after the end of the teens. By the age of twenty or so, the uterus has usually built up strong enough muscles to do a better job.

Third, it is not normal to have cramps continue after the first pregnancy. Labor and delivery really do give the uterus a workout, and this workout increases its efficiency at a tremendous rate.

Fourth, it is better in some ways to have cramps than not to, because cramps are usually an indication that ovulation has taken place. And since ovulation is necessary for full feminine functioning, cramps may be taken as one bit of proof that nature is readying the woman for the job of conception.

Yet normal or not, and helpful or not, cramps are not imaginary. They can be relieved. Doctors usually recommend short bed rests, simple drugs like aspirin, and soothing baths. By soothing baths, doctors mean baths that are neither too hot nor too cold. A significant number of women, although a small percent of the population, suffer from dysmenorrhea—incapacitating cramps thought to be caused by higher than average amounts of prostaglandins. For these women, aspirin and the like will not bring relief. Ponstel and Motrin, which must be prescribed by your doctor, are now recommended for treatment.

The New York psychiatrist Dr. Emy Metzger tells of her experience on the staff of a mental hospital in Vienna in the days when there were no tranquilizers or other soothing drugs for disturbed patients, so they had to be kept in tubs of warm water instead. When their menstrual periods arrived, it was expected that these patients would become even more disturbed and they were taken out of the tubs. "Bathing has been considered unfit for menstruating women since time immemorial, and it is the first rule of medicine to do no deliberate harm," argued the doctors who took them out. But Dr. Metzger suggested leaving them in, at least for a trial. To everyone's astonishment, the warm water helped; they felt better in every way.

The old idea that baths were to be forbidden during menstrual periods was based on the fact that in ancient times most bathing was done in public pools or streams, and it wasn't so much that the water would harm the women as upset the men who dreaded this particular kind of blood. But now that baths are taken in private, and especially now that we know this blood is not dangerous, the taboo no longer makes sense.

And if a soothing bath is not available, an electric pad or warm water bottle may also be helpful, though it should be placed at the feet, not on the abdomen as is commonly done. Heat placed directly on the abdomen can make the uterine squeezes come even faster, and the whole idea is to slow them down.

Things doctors say never to do for cramps are to use opiates, or to stay in bed for several days.

Opiates like codeine, or a barbiturate such as phenobarbital, can be extremely habit-forming, as well as lowering the pain threshold. The more they are used, the less tolerance there is to any pain when they are stopped.

And as for long bed rests, a Philadelphia study divided a large number of girls suffering from cramps into two groups. One group stayed in bed for several days, the other took exercise including vigorous sports like basketball. In the second group, the pain disappeared in half the time.

All doctors agree that the old idea that menstrual pain is caused by a "tipped uterus," that is, a uterus that happens to lie slightly at an angle instead of flat, has gone with the wind. A tipped uterus has no more to do with cramps than a tipped nose. So the insertion of a pessary to try and change its position also makes little sense.

Suppression of Ovulation

If the cramps are bad to the point of being unbearable, doctors usually try to suppress ovulation. They use hormones to do this, usually the ones similar to those in the Pill.

The hormones used are estrogen, progesterone, or a combination of both, and they are given *outside* the normal rhythm. That is, more hormones are given during the first half of the month than would naturally be made by the body, to "stop" the pituitary before it can cause the ovary to release an egg. And without the release of an egg, a two-layer lining that is sometimes difficult for a uterus to expel is not made.

Doctors suppress ovulation for only a short time, though, because sex hormones cause an increase in the size and power of the uterus that is often just enough to tide an adolescent over; she soon gets to the point where she can expel any amount of lining with ease.

Middle Pain

Now to "middle pain."

The Germans called middle pain *mittelschmerz,* and that's what it is—a short, sharp pain that comes during the middle of the cycle rather than during the flow. Middle pain is worrisome because it doesn't seem related to anything. But it is related; it is related to ovulation. Middle pain is a pain in one of the ovaries as an egg bursts forth.

The vast majority of women have no idea that ovulation is taking place unless they take their temperature and notice that it has dropped about half a degree. A few women know about it through this quick pain. Still, women get worried about it because they think the pain may also mean something like appendicitis or other abdominal trouble. If they keep a diary, and note that the pain comes at almost the same time each month, the worry is gone.

Once it is gone, however, doctors suggest that the diary be discontinued. It is not wise to keep looking for any kind of pain since, people being what they are, looking for pain can help bring it on. It's like feeling the dentist's drill in your mouth before he has started, or getting seasick before the boat has left the dock.

TOO LITTLE FLOW OR TOO MUCH

Women also worry if they think they flow too seldom, too frequently or too irregularly. They even worry if they flow every twenty-eight days, but not every twenty-eight days "on the dot."

This should be said in headlines: *No woman flows every twenty-eight days on the dot*. She can flow from twenty-one to forty days apart and still be within the normal range. What is more, she can on occasion skip a cycle completely.

Dr. L. B. Arey says that the average adult woman can expect a third of her periods to vary two or more days from her own expected times, and occasionally very much more.

He sums up his findings this way: "The woman whose periods occur with precise regularity is a creature out of a fairy story. She simply doesn't exist."

NERVOUS CONTROL

One reason that menstrual periods can vary so much is that the glands that control the hormonal waves are affected by the nerves. Because of these nervous influences, any kind of stress can upset the timing—even something so comparatively mild as the stress of an ocean voyage or a change of climate. And strong stresses like fear or anger can upset the periods far more. Fear of pregnancy, for instance, can delay a period just when a woman desires it most; but let her take a test that proves she is not pregnant, and the fear disappears and the period arrives.

Similarly, fear can bring on an unwanted period. Nervous brides often fix a wedding date on which they are sure they will not be menstruating. The day arrives and they find they are flowing anyway.

Dr. Helene Deutsch tells an interesting story about the power of fear or anger to bring on a period out of its usual time. In her book *The Psychology of Women* she tells this tale:

Many years ago, as a young medical student, I followed with great interest a court case concerning a marriage problem. A husband had asked for a divorce and as his only reason told the court the following story. By profession he was a travelling salesman who returned home only at irregular intervals. In the preceding two years, he said, every time he returned home he found his wife menstruating. In his eyes this was sufficient proof that she no longer wished to have marital relations with him even though she assured him in all sincerity that it was only a coincidence, a kind of bad luck for which she was not responsible. The psychiatrists rejected the husband's theory, even though it was already well known that menstruation can exert a tremendous influence upon psychological life. They were ready to admit that mood-changes could accelerate or retard menstruation for a short period, but the enormous and recurrent influence described to them by the husband seemed to these experts impossible. The only person ready to accept the husband's interpretation was the old judge, who had a keen intuition and a broad knowledge of human nature. He granted the divorce, and subsequent events proved the husband's theory to be correct.

As to cramps, there are the stories of the girl who never had them until she became a nurse and had her first brush with the shattering experience of death, and of the girl who had cramps only when falling in and out of love.

ABILITY TO FUNCTION

Because of the endless things that nerves can do to the menstrual periods, and because there are women who have their periods only three or four times a year, Dr. E. C. Hamblen of Duke University bases his definition of normality on the ability to function. He puts it this way: "Any woman who can bear a child is basically normal no matter how much pain she occasionally has, or how often or seldom her periods appear."

Dr. Milton E. J. Senn of Yale expresses this thought in a different way: "The number of variations within the normal is tremendous. This makes our work, when we are dealing with human beings, very difficult and complex. In deciding whether something is pathological or not, we must make sure we are not falling into the error of disregarding human differences. In dealing with the human being, we must be aware of his similarities in comparing him with others, but also be aware of the pitfall of considering someone deviant merely because he is different. His difference may not be unusual for *him*."

Dr. Senn is a pediatrician, and he was writing mainly about children. But his words have such a direct bearing on women that the last sentence is also worth repeating. "The difference may not be unusual for him, or her."

ABSENCE OF MENSTRUATION

Obviously, a woman cannot bear a child if she never menstruates at all, because with no menstruation there is no ovulation, and without ovulation that vital egg is not available to be fertilized. Yet there are girls and women who flow for years, then suddenly stop.

This sudden stopping may be due to several reasons. One is malnutrition. When a girl is seriously undernourished, either as a result of eating next to nothing in an effort to keep her weight abnormally low, or as a result of eating mainly a junk food diet like pickles, potato chips, and fudge sundaes, she can stop menstruating simply because she is not getting enough vitamins to keep herself in good health. Women in concentration camps often stopped for this reason. In her book, *The Walls Came Tumbling Down*, Henriette Roosenburg told of her near starvation in a concentration camp, and how she and almost all the other women there stopped menstruating, losing their sex-desire as well.

Malnutrition can also delay the start of the periods. Right after the First World War in Vienna, when conditions were very bad, seventy-three percent of the girls between fourteen and fifteen years had not started. A few years later, when conditions were much better, only twenty-four percent of the same age group were in the same spot.

Other studies show that girls from better-fed groups start as a rule two years younger than those from undernourished groups. And in the sixteenth and seventeenth centuries, when health conditions in general were terrible, a survey of medical records shows that girls started way behind the early Greeks and Romans who lived better in many ways.

In America today, with probably the best nutrition standards in the history of the world, girls are starting earlier and earlier all the time—much earlier than in Asia and South America. It used to be believed that girls in hot climates started earlier than girls in temperate or cold climates. Not so. Food and health seem to play a more important role.

Psychic Reasons

Other reasons for an absence of flow are emotional, such as a rebellion against femininity.

Some adolescent girls continue to rebel against becoming females. They may rebel consciously or unconsciously, but they rebel just the same. They see growing-up and becoming brides or mothers as something vaguely "dreamy" and "romantic," but suppress what they consider the "disgusting" part. A few repress it so strongly they stop developing and retreat to the stage of infancy, where they eat almost constantly the way a baby does, and become very fat. The fat further hampers their development, since it keeps them from a normal amount of dating.

When such girls begin to eat more sensibly, and especially when they can be led to face both the pleasant and unpleasant parts of growing-up, this often brings on the menstruation that had been suppressed.

Acceptance

As the years go by, the normal woman comes to accept menstruation philosophically. She is not unduly worried when an occasional period is delayed. She is not unduly upset if she has her periods as often as every twenty-one days or as seldom as forty days, since these are within the normal range.

Above all, she comes to accept her periods as a bother, yet seldom more. A bother, but not lastingly painful. A bother, but not "unclean." A bother, but not poisonous to anyone. A bother, but indicating mainly she is at low tide.

Yes, a bother—and a bit of a mess. But accepting mess is one of the signs of maturity. For what isn't a bit of a mess at times, including many experiences that lead through suffering to pleasure? Isn't cooking a meal messy, but doesn't it lead to the pleasure of eating? Isn't washing one's hair or putting on make-up messy, but don't they lead to the pleasure of looking well?

In her novel *The Rosemary Tree* Elizabeth Goudge tells of a precocious five-year-old who was asked by her mother how she always managed to get so dirty.

"I just live," the little girl replied. "Living is dirty work, but I like it."

Menstruation too is sometimes unpleasant. But women learn, if not actually to like it, at least to accept it for what it is, the badge of femininity. The badge can be worn in misery or in pride. It is normal to stress the misery at first, then have it give way to pride—pride in the fact it gives a woman the ability to do what no man can do, bring forth new life.

Norman Mailer confesses to such envy of women that in his book *The Prisoner of Sex* he practically explodes: ". . . somewhere in the insane passions of all men is the huge desire to drive forward into the seat of creation, grab some part of that creation in the hands . . . For man is alienated from the nature which brought him forth; he is not like woman in possession of an inner space which gives her link to the future so he must drive to possess it; he must if necessary come close to blowing his head off that he may possess it."

Would he drive so hard to possess it if he didn't think it a pearl of great price?

5

Women Have Male Hormones Too

When you were born the doctor took a good look at you, gave you the traditional spank on your buttocks, and announced, "It's a boy" or "It's a girl" as the case happened to be.

He was quite definite on the subject. You were one or the other and no mistake.

Your mother was equally definite. She dressed you in pink or blue, and was quite insulted when kind friends, chucking you under the chin in your carriage, murmured, "Isn't he cute?" or "Isn't she adorable?" taking you for the gender you weren't. "He isn't a he, he's a she," she'd explain firmly as she plumped up your pillows. Or, "That's a boy—can't you tell?"

Your mother and doctor made their decisions on one piece of evidence—your obvious sex organs. They looked no further than that. But modern science has looked further, and made the following discovery as a result: There's no such thing as a one hundred percent woman or man.

Your obvious sex organs determine which sex you belong to, but you don't belong to that sex wholly. For almost as important as your outward and visible *organs* are your inward and invisible hormones, and each sex has hormones of the opposite or complementary kind.

A woman has a lot of male hormones. A man has a lot of female hormones. Male hormones are male simply because a man has more of them. Female hormones are female simply because a woman has more of these. But neither one has them exclusively; the absolute he-man is a myth.

Maleness and femaleness are relative. Just as scientists believe the clouds contain both positive and negative electricity which hold them together, so too we are carved from one master mold and each of us contains some positive and negative elements that make us whole.

Centuries ago people had an inkling that this might be true. Long before X-rays or microscopes or chemical laboratories were ever thought of, people looked at a man and were puzzled by certain things they saw. Why, in addition to his large and definite male organ, the penis, did he also have small female nipples and miniature female breasts? Why, in addition to her large and definite female organ, the vagina, did a woman also have a miniature penis or clitoris—the tiny organ near the entrance to the vagina which can become quite erect?

They were equally puzzled by the emotional mystery: Why was a man not entirely "masculine," that is, aggressive, forward, and brave? Why was he also gentle and kind? And why was a woman not exclusively "feminine," that is, gentle and loving? Why was she also aggressive and brave?

This all greatly stirred thoughtful people. And when scientists got to investigating human beings more thoroughly, this is what they found: All normal men have a great deal of the female hormone, or estrogen, and all normal women have a great deal of the male hormone, or androgen.

When the male hormone was discovered it took its name from the Greek word *andros* or "man." But the word androgen isn't actually any more accurate than the word hormone. Just as hormone means literally "to arouse" though hormones also calm down, so does androgen mean literally "the stuff that makes a man" when it makes a woman too.

Both Hormones are Present
Even Before Birth

Even more interesting, scientists found that not only do grown men and women have both kinds of sex hormones, but both kinds are present before birth.

You always thought sex was fixed permanently and irrevocably at the moment of conception? Well, so did everybody else. But no. During the first few weeks after conception the fetus has sex organs that are not yet ovaries or testicles, but may become either as events turn out. In addition, the fetus has two complete sets of Fallopian tubes—one pair male and one pair female, while the external sex organs are little buds that may develop either way.

But after a few weeks the fetal pituitary begins to decide matters, based on the chromosomal makeup of the fetus. If the fetus is to be female, the various glands begin to make more estrogens than androgens. And pushed on by this extra estrogen, the tiny sex-organs become ovaries instead of testes; the female Fallopian tubes expand and develop while the male tubes shrink to nothing; and the little bud on the outside begins to turn inward and become a vagina, making the baby a recognizable Susie instead of a Tom by the time she is born.

But if the embryo is Tom instead of a Susie? Then the opposite takes place. Now the glands make more androgen than they do estrogen—but again only more. The specks become definite testes; the testicles usually descend into the scrotum; and the little bud of a clitoris grows outward until a penis is formed. By the time Tom makes his grand entrance, he has a fine, full set of male organs.

But in both instances the lesser organs do not completely vanish. Susie has her tiny clitoris or miniature penis and Tom has his token breasts.

More, all normal people are born with a large amount of these complementary hormones—so large as to be quite surprising. And not only do we all have a lot of complementary hormones, but women have much more androgen in proportion to their estrogen than men have estrogen in proportion to their androgen. Women, in other words, tend hormonally to be more "masculine" than men to be "feminine." And this larger amount of androgen in women has an important role to play when the menopause comes.

Interestingly, too, brunette women seem to have more male

hormones than blondes. Masculinity, of course, stands for aggression, and Nina Katherine Lunn undoubtedly had this in mind when she remarked: "Perhaps that old joke that 'men prefer blondes but marry brunettes' is founded on this fact of hormone balance. Naturally, if a brunette is more aggressive, she gets her man."

But blonde or brunette, light or dark, tall or short, all women have androgen. And that's the thing that counts.

WHAT DO THE COMPLEMENTARY HORMONES DO FOR US?

Aside from aggression, what do the complementary hormones do for us? What do we have them for?

One important reason is strength. Androgen in both men and women is first and foremost the strength hormone. It maintains and increases body weight. It stimulates growth. It makes for stronger muscles, stronger bones, a stronger body all around. Eunuchs or castrated men aren't so much effeminate as muscularly weakened. With most of their androgens gone, they have lost a prime source of their strength—much more than Samson did when he lost his luxurious hair.

Indeed the effect of androgen on strength is so marked that the late Dr. A. A. Loeser of London, England, made it a practice to give a few injections of androgen to his women patients for several days after a hysterectomy. He did this to increase their muscle tone and ward off fatigue.

Dr. Loeser also extended the same helping hand to a premature baby. A baby born in the ordinary course of events arrives with a relatively high concentration of sex hormones. But a premature baby is apt to be deficient in them. So, to stimulate metabolism and bring about a quick buildup, Dr. Loeser gave such a baby, whether it was a boy or girl, some androgen shots.

Other doctors give them to adolescent boys who aren't growing as fast as they should. I knew one such boy named Bill. Bill at fourteen was puny and undersized—a dumpy boy with a broad body and short legs. Bill was the same at fifteen. But at sixteen, after a few months of androgen treatment, he was tall and well formed—hardly the same lad.

Androgen is the Prime Sex-drive Hormone

Then androgen in men and women is the prime sex-drive hormone. Estrogen gives some sex drive. Androgen gives more. That is why, as you'll see later, the loss of ovaries is comparatively unimportant to a woman as far as her sex life is concerned. Even after such a drastic operation as a total hysterectomy in which both ovaries are removed, she goes on practically as before. For here her own androgen comes to her rescue in a dramatic way.

ANDROGEN AFFECTS THE HAIR AND SKIN

Androgen also affects the hair and skin.

Do you know someone with thick hair on his chest, his arms, and his legs? He can thank a liberal supply of androgen for that. Though, curiously, the same liberal supply may take the hair off his head. Baldness is now considered an almost purely male characteristic due to an excess of androgen, though most men would rather forego the hair on their heads than forego the other characteristics that go with a liberal androgen supply. Eunuchs, on the other hand, have often lost so much of their androgen that they hardly have to shave.

As to the effect of androgen on the skin, doctors now think a relative excess of androgen may be the cause of the famous "adolescent acne" that annoys young boys and girls so much. It isn't that adolescents have too much androgen; rather they get it too quickly. The quick onrush is for a time more than their skins can stand, so John and Helen and Henry get a raft of pimples around sixteen. But as these same people grow into adulthood and their body learns to take care of the increased supply, the pimples usually disappear of their own accord.

ANDROGEN BURNS FAT

Of special interest to you as a woman is the fact that androgen seems to burn fat. The eunuch who gets fat and flabby bears witness to this. And it works, too, the other way around: When the fat, flabby eunuch is given androgen, he regains much of his former muscle tone and masculine form.

On the other hand, women with a high natural androgen count tend to be lean and muscular. We all know women of the superathletic type. An extra supply of androgen may be the cause here.

Estrogen is the Softener

If androgen is the strength giver and hardener, estrogen is the softener. Estrogen in both men and women softens and nourishes. It softens the skin; it nourishes the bones. Do you know some women who all their lives keep a beautiful skin? They can thank a bountiful estrogen supply.

So it all becomes a question of proportion. A large proportion of androgen inclines us one way; of estrogen another. And this proportion changes throughout life. But every last one of us is a blend of male and female hormones; as if we were dipped originally from one great mold and differed only in degree rather than in kind.

NO CONNECTION WITH HOMOSEXUALITY

By now this question must surely have come to your mind: Do the complementary hormones explain homosexuality? Does, for instance, the possession of a larger-than-usual amount of estrogen turn the love instincts of a man toward his own sex?

As far as we know, the answer is "no."

A few years ago, to be sure, doctors thought the answer might be "yes." When the complementary hormones were discovered, doctors hoped they had the answer to homosexuality—a problem that has baffled people since the days of the ancient Greeks. "We'll give a homosexual man a few shots of androgen," they said, "and sit back and await the results."

But the results did not pan out as expected. On the contrary, instead of turning the sex drive of such a man toward a woman, it merely intensified the *same* drive he had already—that is, the one toward men. He became more potent, surely, but the direction of his potency wasn't changed a bit.

At present, then, doctors feel that homosexuality is the result more of psychological than physical factors. At any rate, there's no doubt about it: Some of the most masculine-appearing men are homosexual. Some of the most feminine-appearing men are heterosexual. And ditto with lesbians. Neither appearance nor hormone count seems to be the determining factors as far as we know.

WHERE DO THESE COMPLEMENTARY HORMONES COME FROM?

Another question must also have come to your mind: Where do these complementary hormones come from? What is their source within us? Where do we get them?

Here you may be in for a surprise. A woman gets some androgen from her own ovaries. Yes, that most "feminine" of organs, the ovary, is the source of some androgens as well. And it works similarly in a man. A man gets some estrogens from that most "masculine" of organs, his testes. Indeed, not only do pregnant mares make estrogen, but the greatest source is that extremely masculine animal, a stallion! A stallion like Man o' War or Secretariat creates from four to five hundred times as much estrogen as does the normal woman, and some of it comes from his testes, the same testes that supply his sperm.

But the most surprising source of complementary hormones is a gland that you wouldn't ordinarily associate with sex activity of any kind. I refer here to your adrenal or emergency glands.

Your adrenals are your emergency glands surely. But in a sense they are like the once-famous Two-in-One shoe polish—two glands in one. One part of your adrenals, the medulla, functions in the emergency role. Another part functions as a true sex gland. Indeed the sex function of the medulla of the adrenals is so striking that Dr. A. A. Loeser placed it right up with the ovaries and testes, and refered to the adrenals as "the third sex gland."

As you will see in the next chapter, the adrenals play a sex role throughout your life, making the puzzle of the menopause begin to fit together at last.

6

The Wisdom of Your Body

Walter Cannon was a determined man.

This quiet Harvard professor wasn't satisfied with the experiments that resulted in his great book *Bodily Changes in Pain, Hunger, Fear and Rage.* He was constantly planning new experiments—experiments he hoped would help solve one of the basic mysteries of life: How do we manage to stay alive?

We seem to be made of such unstable stuff! Our ears are jolted by sounds so faint no instrument can catch them. Our noses are set quivering by smells so delicate we can detect one part of, say, vanilla in ten million parts of air. Our eyes are set blinking by light so faint the fastest photographic plate can barely catch it. If we stop breathing for only a few minutes, we die.

What makes this highly unstable stuff of which the human body is composed keep swinging back to stability again?

What Cannon found was a margin of safety—a margin of safety that works in everyday life.

Our "Margin of Safety"
in Everyday Life

When a good dressmaker plans a dress, she buys her material generously, allowing for large seams and a deep hem in case the dress has to be let out later.

When a wise engineer plans a bridge, he designs it to carry

far more than the load he thinks it now must carry. He plans every beam and support to be three, six, even twenty times as strong as necessary. In this way future trucks and crowds of people far heavier than he ever dreamed of can cross it unafraid.

The dressmaker calls her wise planning "foresight." The engineer calls his "allowing for a margin of safety."

Dr. Cannon found that our bodies have this margin of safety too. We are cunningly put together to take on almost anything that may come along.

When light gets too bright for our eyes to bear it, this margin of safety goes to work. We automatically blink, thus resting our eyes for a second. This rest enables us to take up the job of seeing again.

When a foreign particle enters our eyes, we automatically produce tears. These tears bathe our eyes and help carry the particle away.

When air for breathing gets scarce, we gasp. This gasping causes extra air to rush into our lungs faster than usual.

When we cut a finger and are threatened with the loss of a lot of blood, the blood, that might otherwise have flowed out too quickly, soon clots. In this way, except in the case of rare people, such as "bleeders," the flow is automatically stopped.

Then look at the wonderful way we keep our internal temperatures stabilized. How much better off we are in the matter of temperatures than, say, the frog. Our normal temperature is 98.6° F. We keep coming back to it as a rule come what may. But not the frog. When the outside temperature drops, a frog gets as cold as the weather and must sink to the bottom of a pond and stay there motionless all winter long. Yet the thermometer can drop to forty below; by a cunning arrangement we stick to our 98.6° F. nevertheless.

How do we do it? Mainly by shivering. We automatically shiver, which causes a motion which warms us up. We also get "goose-pimples," and these contract the skin and send the blood rushing to our warmer insides. The same goose-pimples cause the tiny hairs on our arms and legs to stand upright, making these hairs trap a little blanket of air within them, which further warms us up; while really intense cold causes a special rush of adrenal hormones to pour out into our bloodstream. This adrenal rush acts like opening the dampers of a furnace. We get heated up now doubly quick.

And if we get too hot instead of too cold? Why, then, we do just the opposite—we perspire and evaporate away some of the excess heat. Theoretically, the heat produced inside a woman by such an ordinary job as scrubbing a floor should be enough to cook some of her tissues as hard as a hard-boiled egg. But, the "margin of safety" comes to the rescue once more. The harder she works, the more she perspires, and she returns again to that 98.6° F.

THAT MARGIN OF SAFETY IN ILLNESS

Safety factors such as these protect us in everyday life. But what about emergencies? Really great crises? Do similar factors come to our rescue here? Dr. Cannon probed some more.

Surely tuberculosis was for centuries a major crisis of the body. But when a man had to have one lung collapsed, the other lung carried on almost as well without it. The margin of safety here is thus one hundred percent.

Next he considered kidney disease, another great emergency. Here he found the safety margin to be about equally as great. A man can lose as much as two thirds of both kidneys yet still suffer no serious disturbance as a result.

And finally he considered the parts of the body that are not in pairs like the lungs and the kidneys. What happened when a man has to lose most of his stomach? Or his wife her gall bladder? Seemingly irreplaceable parts like those?

Well, here there is an even more remarkable adjustment. When one part of the body is knocked out of the picture, a totally different part sometimes takes its place! You have a margin of safety far beyond your needs.

In 1932 Walter Cannon published another book, *The Wisdom of the Body*. This book contains a great message of hope:

that from imbalance we tend to swing back to balance, from instability to stability, from disturbance to rest.

THE MENOPAUSE HAS ITS OWN WISDOM OF THE BODY

By good fortune Cannon's principles apply to a woman in her menopause.

In the menopause the "margin of safety" works so that, as you pass through your changing time, you will find that as one part of your gland system moves out, another moves in.

Let's look a little more closely now at what is happening to you during that time, and you'll see why this is so.

How THE MENOPAUSE STARTS:
THE NORMAL PATTERNS

The word menopause means literally "the pausing of the monthly process."

If you want to be strict about it, the word refers to the actual moment at which menstruation stops. But that moment comes so differently to different women that the whole changing time is usually referred to as the menopause, rather than any particular month.

How does the menopause start? How will you know when you are entering it? That's a little hard to tell. If we were all peas in a pod, it might come to us in the same way. But since we are individuals, there is no one pattern for all.

However, there are three main patterns, each of them perfectly normal. Any of these may be yours:

Normal pattern one: This is the easiest, and the one women pray for, but alas seldom get. In this pattern, the flow remains the same, but one fine day it just up and disappears all at once and doesn't come back.

Normal pattern two: This is the next easiest. Now instead of disappearing all at once, the flow gradually gets lighter and lighter each month. But at last it, too, disappears for good.

Normal pattern three: This is the most puzzling and annoying of the lot. The flow stops and starts again with a light flow interspersed with a heavy flow. In addition, the flows sometimes come more frequently than before, that is, much less than a month apart. For what seems like forever, they keep you all at sea until finally they, too, disappear.

To repeat: All of the above patterns are normal. None of them should cause you either worry or alarm.

THE ABNORMAL PATTERNS

There are also abnormal patterns that should cause concern. These patterns are:

Abnormal pattern one: A flow that *persistently* appears more frequent than usual—say, every two weeks or so.

Abnormal pattern two: A flow that gets heavier and heavier every month with no light flow between.

Abnormal pattern three: The appearance of unexplained blood immediately after sexual intercourse or after using a vaginal douche.

Abnormal pattern four: A flow that comes back, not just after two or three months but a full six months after you have not flowed at all. Especially if it comes back when you have not been taking hormone pills of any kind.

Any of these abnormal patterns call for an immediate checkup. And by checkup I mean an examination by a gynecologist. This is no time for a hurried consultation with the corner druggist or your best bosom friend. And it certainly is no time to save money for a new winter coat instead of seeing a doctor at all.

In fact, even when the pattern is normal, a checkup and Pap test twice a year is something you owe yourself at this time in your life. Remember, you're an important person. It's far nicer to go to a doctor regularly during the changing years and hear what Dr. I. C. Fischer of Mt. Sinai Hospital in New York likes to say to his patients—"Just a slight case of menopause"—than to delay and hear something with a much more solemn sound.

Something else: During the changing years you should keep a diary. Get a small one and tuck it in your purse. Then every time a menstrual period arrives, make an entry of the date. Make another careful entry of the date it stops as well. Equally important, put down how often you change your napkins or tampons each day.

Because if you do have to go see a doctor, the first question he'll be sure to ask you is, "Are they heavy or light flows that are coming now?" And the only way he can judge heavy or light with reasonable accuracy is according to how many napkins or tampons you use. While as for the length of time between periods and the number of days each lasts, it's bad enough to try to remember these during the more regular times of your life, much less when they may be bouncing around.

But if you keep a calendar or diary instead of thinking out loud, "Let's see—my last period was the day of the Church Bake Sale—— Oh no, it wasn't, it was the day the Bridge Club met," you'll *know*. And knowing will not only help your doctor, it will help reassure you that your menopause is probably arriving in a more normal way than you think.

Your Ovaries Step Off the Seesaw

But in whatever way it arrives, whether normally or abnormally (and to the vast majority of us it does arrive normally), it adds up to essentially the same thing: your ovaries are stepping down from the glandular balance-scale.

Your ovaries, as you now know, have been on that seesaw for many years, balancing your chief gland in a monthly fall and rise. Over and over again this monthly game has been played. First your pituitary has been on the up end of the saw, signaling your ovaries to "go!" Then your ovaries have been on the up end, signaling your chief gland to "stop!"

Around the age of fifty that fine stop-and-go arrangement is interrupted. It is interrupted for the simple reason that your ovaries are stepping down.

The age of fifty as a stepping-down age is of course strictly average. I stress that because women worry if the changing years don't happen exactly then. But it is not too unusual for menstruation to depart of its own accord as early as thirty-five. And in rare cases it has been known to continue until sixty-five or beyond. Nor does the fact that you started to menstruate early mean that you will stop early. Or started late, stop late. People used to think that, but now it seems that it works just the other way round. The newest experiments indicate that if you started *early,* you are apt to stop *late.* It looks as if nature had selected a certain group of women as especially fitted for childbearing and given them a longer menstrual span.

At any rate, around the age of fifty the flow of most women begins to depart. And along with the flow, fertility departs too. Occasionally, to be sure, an egg may slip through and become fertilized. Women have been known to conceive as long as a full year after menstruation has ceased. But in general this does not happen. As a rule, when menstruation goes, fertility goes too.

After many years of work, your ovaries are now completing their life task. They are stepping down from their place on the balance-scale. This stepping down of your ovaries is one of the main clues to the puzzle of the menopause. It's a main clue because, without your ovaries to balance it, your chief gland is left high and dry in midair. The ovarian hormone tide that used to shoot up each month and bring it down again is simply shooting up no more.

But—and this is an important *but*—your chief gland does not immediately realize your ovaries are stepping down. On the contrary, like a too conscientious workman who does not know the bell has rung, your pituitary actually works away harder than ever, trying to stir up a pair of ovaries that progressively fail to respond.

It is this combination of a too persistent pituitary and progressively failing ovaries that causes the trouble. This, as far as we know, is the reason for the upsets of the menopause when such upsets occur.

Frustrated at getting erratic responses and finally no response from your ovaries, your pituitary sometimes sends frantic messages to your thyroid instead. And these frantic messages can throw your whole hormone system out of balance; throw your whole nervous system out of balance; throw the whole *you* out of balance and shake you from top to toe.

Your Adrenals May Take Over

But here's another clue: these upsets are usually temporary. Within a short time your "margin of safety" usually starts to work. And in this case your safety factor is none other than your adrenal glands, because what sometimes happens now is this: Your adrenals come to your rescue in one of their emergency roles.

As your ovaries make estrogens in gradually decreasing amounts, your adrenals sometimes start to make both estrogens and androgens in gradually increasing amounts. These increased adrenal hormones in time take over some of the old jobs of the ovarian hormones and quiet down your hormone system.

So if you have a normal menopause, as most of us do, you can expect that the new sex hormones from your adrenals will partly compensate for the old sex hormones from your ovaries. In this way the scale will be quieted; a new balance will be achieved.

Or, to paraphrase Cannon's beautiful words: The wisdom of your body will see you through.

How Your Doctor Can Help You

If your body comes around to this new state of balance of its own accord, why then do some women suffer from things like flushes, nervousness, headaches, and fatigue? Why does anyone ever get some of those?

The answer is: Your body is a God-given machine. It can do what no man-made machine can do—repair itself. But this repair takes time. The seesaw will right itself, but maybe not so quickly or so completely as you might wish.

And while it is righting itself, a "learning period" may be necessary while you are getting used to the new state of affairs. Just as a learning period was necessary during adolescence when you had to get used to a greatly increased supply of sex hormones, so it may also be necessary while you are getting used to a decreased supply. And during this learning period you may need help.

Meanwhile you may be in for discomfort for several months or, in extreme cases, several years. Not all women have discomfort, to be sure. Estimates differ as to how many do and how many do not. But an outstanding authority like Dr. Emil Novak of Baltimore, Maryland, says that no more than about thirty-five percent of all women have menopausal trouble or pain of any kind. According to Dr. Novak, the other sixty-five percent of us learn our new role so quickly that we hardly know any change is taking place.

This sixty-five percent who have an uneventful menopause

may be like Emily Nathan of Cincinnati. Emily is a tall, red-haired woman who set out on a hunting trip to Canada with her husband Lou. When they got to Montreal, which was to be their last stopping place before setting out for the wilds, Emily said: "How about staying here in the hotel a few days longer, Lou? Come to think of it, my menstrual period is due any day now. And if we stay here I can get it over and done with, and have almost a whole clear month." Lou agreed, and they waited. They waited a week. They waited two weeks. They might have been waiting yet, because Emily never did menstruate again nor has she to this day, three years later. Without any discomfort whatever Emily had joined the happy sixty-five percent. The menopause had arrived for her with never a sign.

YOU MAY BE AS FORTUNATE AS THAT

There's every chance you may be among the fortunate group. Why not? No crystal-gazer can possibly tell in advance who will be among them and who won't. Women who have been "weak" all their lives often become stronger than they expect. Women who have been "strong" may find that they do not have the strength they once had. Even the fact that your mother had a hard time means nothing. Heredity plays little part here. In fact, Dr. Earl T. Engle of New York's Columbia Presbyterian Hospital tells of a whole town in New Hampshire where not one single woman had a bit of difficulty. In that town there was not even one menopausal twinge.

But if you're not in the fortunate group, if you're in the other thirty-five percent instead, then you may have anything from a mild upset to downright pain. Oddly, too, these discomforts may sometimes not arrive with the menopause itself, but come a long time after menstruation has completely stopped. This happened to a friend of mine, Helen Carter, a Brooklyn department store executive. Helen had no trouble for several years after the start of her menopause, then she had a few months of real discomfort. Since nobody had told her this might happen, she was quite bewildered for a time.

SOME OF THE DISCOMFORTS AND PAINS

Here, then, are some of the discomforts and pains that you may have. They may arrive either while you are still menstruating, during the time it is subsiding, or when it has totally stopped.

Most women do not experience more than a few of them. You haven't a chance in a million of getting the whole list. And even with those you do get, there will often be long intervals of freedom and peace.

The Hot Flushes or Flashes

The hot flushes or flashes get first mention. They do so by sheer weight of bad reputation, for no one can deny that the flushes are the most famous and the most exasperating of changing time experiences.

They're exasperating because some women get so many of them—up to dozens a day. And as for their fame, they've been talked about so much that the word "flushes" is almost linked with the word "menopause" as butter is with bread. I even knew a man who parodied the famous cola ad and called it "the menopause that reflashes." He thought he was quite a card!

A hot flush or flash is just about what the name implies—a quick flush of heat that starts at the nipple line and rises up over the neck and face. It is different from an ordinary feeling of heat that is spread all over the body and comes gradually. The flushes come quickly, and are confined mostly to the head and neck.

Flushes may last only a second, and they may last a full minute or more. Dr. John Hannan of London, England, once timed them at an average of thirty seconds. I once had one that lasted ten minutes as I was eating lunch one day. All of a sudden my face got suffused with heat and became all screwed up and twisted while my jaws got stuck so tight I couldn't eat another bite. When I looked in the mirror, I hardly recognized myself, I was so twisted and lined. But just as unexpectedly as it had come, the whole thing vanished. Nor did I ever have another like it.

What causes these flushes or flashes? Nobody exactly knows. The best explanation seems to be your temporary glandular imbalance. Since your glands send messages to each other by way of the bloodstream, when your gland scale is off balance your hormones don't operate smoothly and regularly. Instead they operate in rushes and stops. The rushes dilate the tiny arteries and send a quick spurt of blood to your skin, giving a quick sensation of heat; the stops draw the blood away and give a quick sensation of cold.

Flushes are no more than a nuisance and a vexation to many women. Others find them extremely unpleasant because they make them perspire so freely they are sure everybody notices them. But they have one redeeming feature. Of all menopausal disturbances, the flushes are the easiest to get under control. With proper treatment (which will be discussed later) they can be reduced from many to few.

A Dry, Itching Vagina

A devilish accompaniment of the menopause is a dry, itching vagina. This can be very uncomfortable, especially during or after intercourse.

The sex organs, as you know, are a prime target of estrogen. When estrogen is fading, its loss is felt particularly in the vagina, which becomes thinner and drier over the years. It can become so dry that intense itching may result. If this happens, a simple jelly like KY lubricating jelly, which is tasteless, odorless, and nongreasy, will be a pleasant aid. No prescription is needed for it. (I'll talk about other remedies in a later chapter.)

Crawling Out of Your Skin

A strange accompaniment of the menopause may be the feeling you are crawling out of your skin. A woman I know said she once felt like a snake that was shedding, and was sure this had never happened to anyone else. But when she compared notes with her friends she found they had the same experience, and she felt much relieved.

Gas

Another strange accompaniment can be the development of quite a bit of "gas" that makes the stomach look distended, and no figure-conscious woman wants to look like that.

Dr. William Bickers explains this gas. "As estrogen fails," he says, "the adrenal cortex increases its activity, producing both new estrogens and androgens. This production of new androgens changes the sodium-potassium balance of the blood and encourages the development of gas. I have found the best treatment is to increase the potassium intake. The richest sources of potassium in nature are bananas, tomato juice, and orange juice. These can be further supplemented by the use of a potassium powder dissolved in water."

So if you are greatly disturbed by gas, the moral is plain. Eat a few extra bananas, and drink more tomato and orange juice, the last preferably freshly squeezed. I was given an electric orange squeezer with which to make fresh juice, and what a difference there is in taste. Also, the vitamins in orange juice quickly evaporate when they are exposed to the air or otherwise handled, so you have a double reason for making it fresh.

As for bananas, when I was a child my parents used to say they could put me on a desert island with a bunch of bananas and a case of seltzer water and I would be happy. Then I became worried that bananas were fattening and cut them out—until I found they are roughly the equivalent of a baked potato, so I could substitute one for the other. I find a fine pick-me-up is a glass of skim milk mixed with two tablespoons of a high protein powder you can get in any health-food store. Shake them together or whirl them in a blender with half a banana. Delicious, full of potassium and calcium, and low in calories to boot.

Insomnia

Insomnia comes next. Even those people who normally "sleep like a log" may be plagued for a while by this distress. They may get to sleep in their usual fashion, then wake up with a jolt in the middle of the night as if they were in a car and the driver suddenly stepped hard on the accelerator. Why is this? A sudden momentary rush of blood seems to send a message to your head that shakes you and wakes you up.

But once more the good news is: don't let the insomnia worry you. If you get rid of that bugaboo that loss of sleep drives people out of their minds, and if you can relax and remember the moments of upset will pass, then nine chances to one they *will* pass in a few weeks or months, and your old sleep habits will return.

Also, don't forget that the flushes tend to come much more frequently at night. Indeed, some doctors call them "night sweats." Obviously, they can awaken you from what would otherwise be a sound sleep.

Forgetfulness

A comparatively minor annoyance to some women is the forgetting of small things. Suddenly you can't remember where you put something, or the date of your best friend's birthday. But this happens to everyone. Working women, to whom small details may be very important, seem to notice it more. But when they stop trying to remember, the information often pops into their heads.

Polyuria

Polyuria is a word meaning frequent urination. Polyuria can be annoying indeed. To have constantly to go to the bathroom, especially during the night, is most exasperating.

The cause? Probably your pituitary. Your pituitary regulates the water content of your body. When your pituitary changes its pace, as during the menopause, the water balance of your tissues is disturbed and during the day more water than usual is stored up. Then at night this extra water is released from your tissues into your kidneys. The result is pressure on your bladder and the constant desire to urinate.

Also, lack of estrogen is felt locally in the bladder, just as it is felt locally in the vagina. The opening of the bladder narrows as you age, so you have to go to the bathroom more often, even though less water is passed each time. The dividing line between the vaginal wall and the uterus is very thin at all ages, and as the years pass it may become thinner. All of this contributes to a frequent desire to "go."

Getting back to polyuria. I'm one of those people who, since my college days, have always had to go to the bathroom frequently. When I asked my doctor what to do, he answered simply: "Go!"

Nervousness and Fatigue

Nervousness and fatigue are so generally connected with the changing years that they seem to be linked with them like crackers are linked with cheese.

One woman describes her nervousness this way: "There are days when for no reason I simply feel jumpy all over." Another: "Common street noises that didn't bother me before now sometimes seem to drive me mad."

This state of affairs naturally brings up that old terrible bugaboo: "I must be going out of my mind." This thought is all the more persistent in those women who have no flushes or other menopausal symptoms. To them, the nervousness and irritability seem to spring from nowhere. At least, they do until the women think them out.

The way to think them out is this: During the days just before each menstrual period many women feel depressed and blue due to a low hormone state. Indeed this premenstrual depression is so common the Paris police believe that most female shoplifting and stealing crimes are committed at this time, though other police do not agree with them. The important thing to remember is that the premenstural depression usually passes so quickly you hardly have a chance to notice it. The menopausal depression sometimes lasts longer, so it may make a dent. If you look at it this way, it will not worry you unduly. You will realize that when nature corrects your hormone condition it also will pass.

I remember one Saturday afternoon not long ago, lying on my sofa listening to the Metropolitan Opera broadcast of *Madame Butterfly,* and weeping a regular lake full of tears. I had heard *Madame Butterfly* many times. It is a sad story, but not so sad that I should lie there like a schoolgirl and weep. Weep I did, though, and anyone happening into the room might have thought something awful had happened to me personally. But it was only the woes of poor Cho-Cho-San.

Unnatural? Not at all. Going out of my mind? Not a bit of it. It was only the "menopause blues."

What I should have done was to get out of the house fast, and taken myself to the corner drugstore for a treat like an ice-cream soda. Bad for my figure perhaps. But both the walk and the treat would have been excellent for my morale.

The Tension Headaches That
Seem Like "Brain Pains"

Next after the flushes in nuisance value come the tension headaches. They're next because, while not nearly so common as the flushes, they can be far more unpleasant. For these are not ordinary headaches—the kind that last for an hour or two and are chased by a couple of aspirin. They are what are commonly called "sick headaches"—the kind that sweep through the body from head to toe. They can be accompanied by severe throbbing of the temples, double vision, a stomach going heave-ho, dizziness, and chills. What is more, they may start in the morning and last the entire day, growing progressively worse until finally sleep wears them off.

I was astonished by my first such experience a short time after my ovaries as well as my uterus had been removed in a complete hysterectomy. I had practically never had a headache in my life, but I awoke one morning with this strange, terrible throbbing. I could barely make it from the bed to the bathroom. The light hurt my eyes so much I had to put on dark glasses. I had absolutely no desire to eat.

I couldn't for the life of me figure out what had caused it. "A headache," I said to myself, "is usually caused by something. Some mental strain. Some eye weariness. Some wrong food." But I remembered nothing out of the ordinary. What in thunder could have caused it to start?

When it lasted three whole days, getting progressively worse, I was really stumped. At last it dawned on me that it must have something to do with my hysterectomy. So I staggered to the phone and called the surgeon who had operated on me. He merely barked, "Nonsense—it has nothing to do with the operation," and abruptly hung up.

But he was wrong. It wasn't nonsense, and it had everything to do with it.

Because I had another headache a few weeks later. And another. And another. And since then I have talked to dozens of women who had similar headaches—my mother's hairdresser, my farm neighbor over the hill, the boardinghouse keeper up the road.

I also talked to many doctors, who agreed that headaches may be definitely caused by fluctuating hormone levels, though on the other hand many women who have had headaches all their lives lose them during the menopause.

What can you do about these headaches if you get them? You can recognize them for what they are, and not be panicked by them as I was. You can say to yourself, "They will pass. They will pass." For that is what they will almost surely do, though you may need special medicine to help in the meantime.

That's what has been happening to me. The headaches have been almost my only changing-time trouble, in spite of the fact that a surgical menopause always tends to be worse than a natural one. But even at that they have been gradually disappearing. At the beginning I got them fairly regularly about two weeks apart. Now they disappear and do not return for months. At the beginning they lasted an entire day or more, now they last for an hour or two. Someday I hope I'll have my last one; I will bid them good-bye forever.

Still one other word about the headaches. In almost no case, no matter how bad they are, will they mean "you are going out of your mind," or "something is wrong with your brain." The brain controls pain felt in other parts of the body, but there are no feeling nerves in the brain itself. You could cut a person's brain up into little pieces if you had to and there would be no pain.

Headaches are still quite mysterious. Sometimes they come when the veins in the head fill up with blood, as they can do very quickly, and go away when the blood drains away. Other times they are due to tension and fatigue. Nobody can exactly pinpoint them. But while you may feel utterly miserable the day you have a headache, rest assured your brain will not be damaged in the least.

Pains at the Back of the Neck

Some women who get no headaches get strange pains in the back and sides of the neck. These aren't throbbing pains; they are rather slow and steady. As another farm neighbor of mine, stout Mrs. Williams, described them: "You feel a slow, steady pain that starts in the neck and reaches out and around your shoulders, and sometimes up to the back of your head. When that happens, you feel as if you'd like to unscrew your neck and take your head off for a while and set it down for a rest."

Needless to say, these neck pains have nothing to do with your mind or brain either. There are several important nerves located in your neck, and these are what may be vibrating. If you massage the sides and back of your neck slowly and firmly, it will help a lot.

Pains in the Chest That Seem Like Heart Pains

One queer fact about the menopause is that almost everything about it can seem like something much worse than it is. Just as headaches and neck pains can seem like brain pains but not be, so occasional shooting pains in the chest can seem like heart pains but not be heart pains at all.

Dr. David Scherf says these menopausal chest pains are due to temporary glandular imbalance—the same old imbalance that causes all the other troubles you may have. For some unknown reason, when your ovarian supply is low, these strange chest pains may appear.

But Dr. Scherf has found that even *young* girls with ovarian deficiency get similar chest pains. Yet when these girls are given ovarian hormones to make up for the deficiency, the pains go away. (Of course constant severe chest pains demand an immediate and special investigation, such as an EKG.)

Great Fatigue

During the menopause some women experience great and inexplicable fatigue—inexplicable because it is not ordinary fatigue, the kind that comes after a hard day's work, but rather a strange kind of tiredness. You may start the morning feeling fine and chipper, then suddenly feel as if you can't make it back from the grocery store six blocks away. Or feel like I did one day when I had gone uptown to do some shopping but was suddenly so completely exhausted after only two hours that I almost wanted to sit down on the curbstone. For one awful moment it seemed as if I literally could not stand.

This kind of fatigue may come in waves, too. That is, for a few days you may be fine, then the next few days be so tired all you want to do is sink into a rocker and "set." Then more days or weeks of feeling fine, another few days of being tired, and so on and on. Yet nothing at all except the menopause may be the matter with you.

One woman who objected strenuously to the fatigue was a Massachusetts businesswoman. "I just can't *afford* to be tired. I just can't!" she would wail, until she realized it would pass, and it did.

How Your Doctor Can Help You

Now what can your doctor do to help you? A great deal. Fifty years ago he could do practically nothing. And before that? He could do absolutely nothing. Here, for instance, is a prescription taken from an old medical book of the Renaissance, dated 1491: "To check the irregular flow of a woman in the menopause, give a decoction of myrrh and apples. A cure may sometimes also be effected by pouring some of this same substance into her sandals and urging the patient to walk." Still earlier, during the time of the Greeks, there was the theory of the "wandering womb." Hippocrates explained the theory this way: "that part of a woman which is called the womb, being an animal desirous of generation . . . if it become unfruitful for a long time, turns indignant, and, wandering all over the body, stops the passage of the spirits and the breathing, and occasions the most extreme hysteria and all sorts of diseases." The only thing to be done was to "find" the womb and bring it back where it belonged!

Today a good physician has proven menopausal medicines that can help. These are hormonal medicines and they are among the greatest boons to women of anything ever found. Among them are the estrogens.

Two Kinds of Estrogen

There are two kinds of estrogens, each quite different. You will want to understand this difference because, if you do take them, it may be important to you in the way you react.

The first of these comes from natural sources. It is a boiled down concentrate made from the urine of animals. Just as calves' liver is boiled down and concentrated into a drug to help anemia, so is the urine of animals boiled down and concentrated into an estrogen that helps women through their changing time.

The second kind comes completely from synthetic or chemical sources. It is entirely made in the laboratory.

From your point of view each has certain advantages and disadvantages.

The chemical estrogen has the advantages of being more powerful and much cheaper than that from natural sources. A common one is called stilbestrol, and it comes in seven or eight different strengths. But the rub is that some women can't tolerate the chemical brand. They become nauseated, get hives, or pains in their breasts. These symptoms may wear off after a few days as they build up a tolerance to the medicine. In other women the symptoms don't wear off; they persist. For this reason, few doctors these days recommend chemical estrogen.

The kind boiled down and purified from animal urine is more costly, but practically no one gets upset from it. A well-known estrogen of this kind is called Premarin.

Interestingly, an excellent source of animal estrogen is the urine of the pregnant mare. The mare gives off great quantities of estrogen while she is pregnant; so much so that all over the country there are large horse-breeding farms where mares are kept constantly pregnant in order to give off estrogen for women to use. The name Premarin comes from "pregnant mare's urine."

When I started to take estrogen my husband laughingly referred to it as my "horse medicine." So it was.

MONEY SAVING TIPS

In 1979 the brand-name copyright on Premarin expired, so you can now also get it under the generic name of "conjugated estrogen." Ask your doctor to prescribe it that way. It will save you a lot of money.

Also, many people have difficulty with new medicines, so another money-saving trick I've learned is to get only *part* of a new prescription from the drugstore. If I have a prescription that calls for, say, thirty tablets, I ask the druggist to let me have only half a dozen, then I tell him to keep the prescription on file until I decide if I want the rest. Since there is no drug in the world that agrees with everybody, this has saved me many dollars through the years, not to mention not cluttering up the family medicine chest with stuff that nobody wants or any longer needs.

But whether you pay a few cents a pill or more, estrogen can do a real job for you. It can cut down the number of your flushes from many to few. It can change a dry vagina to a moist one; it can reduce the urge to urinate frequently. It can lessen the fatigue and diminish the nervousness, and do away with some of the insomnia. In short, it can replace your own dwindling hormone supply and make every menopausal symptom easier to bear.

It may not quickly take away all changing-time discomforts, but it will take away so many you'll be grateful indeed.

ESTROGEN BY INJECTION OR BY MOUTH?

Yet we still haven't rounded out the estrogen story.

Is there an advantage to taking estrogen by injection versus taking it by mouth?

When estrogen first burst upon a welcoming world back in

the 1920s, it was given mainly by injection. That was largely because strong, effective pills had not yet been developed. Also, some women seemed to prefer injections because they thought injections had a certain magic quality about them. Or they forgot to take their pills and wanted to rely on a regular visit to a doctor for a shot instead. While still others wanted the reassurance of a chat.

But the injection method usually costs much more than the pill method. Also, all injections have the risk of causing infection. Therefore, some doctors start treatment with long-lasting injections that are slowly released into the body. They usually give only two injections, a month apart, however, then switch to pills.

How Much Estrogen Do You Need?

How much, if any, estrogen do you need? In the old days doctors had to guess, but they can now determine through a test called the Maturation Index test, which is done by examining the cells in a sample of your vaginal secretions.

During your entire life, the appearance of your vaginal cells has been changing, as your estrogen tides have gone up and down. Their appearance has changed during the various days of the menstrual month; it has changed during pregnancy; it changes during the menopause as well. Doctors have therefore discovered that they can take a small sample of your vaginal secretions as easily as they take a sample of your saliva, send this sample to a laboratory where it is studied under a microscope, and learn quite accurately from the subsequent report the state of your estrogen supply, or how "mature" your vaginal cells are.

This Maturation Index test, together with a similar test called the Pap cancer test (named after its creator, the Greek doctor George Papanicolaou) is an immensely helpful guide. When a good doctor treats you during or after the menopause, he will want to see you twice a year, give you a thorough physical exam each time, and determine your estrogen dose accordingly.

Not all doctors do a Maturation test, however. Some do what is called the "finger test." Normally, a woman's vagina has many folds. If it has very few folds, which can be determined by a doctor slipping two of his fingers into the vagina, then you probably need some estrogen. Still others go by the number of flushes you report, and prescribe accordingly.

TAKE NO MORE ESTROGEN THAN YOU NEED

It can't be repeated too often: No woman should take more estrogen than is prescribed. All drugs taken in excess can be harmful; stimulating drugs can be particularly harmful. And estrogen can be so stimulating it can cause all kinds of trouble.

Too much estrogen can overstimulate your breast tissue to the point where your breasts become heavy, sore, and full.

Too much estrogen can bring about a most annoying increase in vaginal secretions.

Too much estrogen can make you put on extra weight due to water retention.

Too much can make you bleed again after your regular periods have stopped, bleed so irregularly your doctor may have to send you to a hospital for a D and C (dilatation and curettage) to make sure nothing serious is wrong.

Above all, too much can cause cancer of the lining of the womb.

Because of this, the rule is: take as little estrogen as possible, and for the shortest length of time. Stop when your truly upsetting symptoms disappear, even if later you have to start again.

Androgens as Medicine

Let's dismiss the estrogens for the time being, and consider the androgens as menopausal medicine.

The androgens, as you know, are the other sex hormones— the "male" hormones always present in both men and women. So when estrogens alone do not work, doctors will use estrogens in combination with androgens.

Dr. A. A. Loeser put his feelings about the matter into these words: "Estrogens are the steady, discreetly working principles. They have the upper hand over the androgens in normal conditions. But if they are greatly in excess, then they should be counteracted by androgenic principles to maintain the female-male ratio."

Dr. Loeser therefore often used a combination of both for his menopausal patients. "The male hormone not only prevents a possible estrogenic bleeding, but acts as a stimulant for the general condition, so that fatigue and many of the nervous symptoms disappear," Dr. Loeser explained.

Dr. William Bickers agrees with Dr. Loeser. He mixes androgen with estrogen almost as a routine.

So if friends of yours who don't know what they are talking about scare you with whispers such as: "Androgens will change you completely," or: "Androgens will make you into a man," answer them with "Nonsense." It can't be repeated often enough that androgens are normal to all women. Ever since the moment you first saw the light of day you've been regularly producing androgens—almost as much as many men. Small doses, far from harming you, may make you feel well and strong again, provided the dose is kept at the proper level for *you*.

However, there are undoubtedly precautions to take while taking androgen, just as there are while taking estrogen, since in all life there are thorns with every rose. Here they are:

1. Too much androgen can cause a lot of unwanted hair to grow.

2. Too much androgen can cause acne.

3. Too much androgen can deepen a woman's voice.

Now the first two are seldom permanent. If androgen should cause a lot of hair to grow, this may disappear as soon as the medicine is stopped.

A little bit of unwanted hair is almost inevitable after the menopause. This is because no matter what you do or don't do, when your estrogen balance goes down, your androgen balance comparatively goes up. And androgen is the hair-growth principle. A little extra amount may be just enough to let a few hairs straggle and show, especially on the face and chin.

The same with acne. Too much androgen may cause acne in

grown women for much the same reason it causes it in adolescents. In adolescence a boy or girl gets a great rush of androgen all at once, and his or her body isn't ready to cope with it. But after a while the body learns how and the acne disappears. And some women are more sensitive to androgen than others. An outbreak of acne means "cut down." The acne will almost certainly disappear.

But the voice change may or may not disappear. Dr. Frank Adair of New York's Memorial Hospital tells of a tiny nurse who had been taking enormous amounts of androgen. She startled everybody by booming through the hospital corridors for the rest of her days in a deep manly voice.

So you don't have to worry about a little extra hair growth or acne if you get it while taking androgen, since in all likelihood it will go away when you cut it down or out. But don't disregard any sign of a voice change. Rush to your doctor like lightning if you find yourself getting hoarse.

Dr. A. A. Loeser summed up the androgen cautions for us in this way: "Minute doses of male hormone stimulate femininity; moderate doses depress femininity; massive doses antagonize it completely."

Thyroid Can Help Too

Thyroid, along with estrogen and androgen, can be still another comfort while you change, if an exam shows it is needed.

Why thyroid? you ask. Isn't thyroid a general energy hormone instead of a sex hormone? Where, then, does thyroid come in?

Well, it comes in for the very reason that it *is* a general energy hormone. Sometimes a general push is what you need. Yet the use of thyroid in the menopause has been largely overlooked.

As Dr. W. H. Stoner argued before the American Pharmaceutical Association: "There is a tendency, since the availability of the high-powered, purified steroid (sex) hormones . . . to use them instead of the lowly, old-fashioned thyroid. It should be kept in mind that thyroid is a stimulant to all the tissues of the body . . . and that frequently better results are obtained by stimulating the deficient gland with small doses of thyroid than by supplying the deficient hormone in substitution therapy."

Or, to put Dr. Stoner's statement more simply: You can sometimes get better results by taking thyroid along *with* the sex hormones. Sometimes by just taking thyroid alone.

Margaret Bates is an example of a woman who was helped by thyroid alone. Margaret is a busy newspaper columnist in Atlanta, Georgia. When she suddenly stopped menstruating at thirty-one, her doctor decided that that was too soon even for an early menopause. So, after tests which showed she needed it, he put her on thyroid. No hormones of any other kind were used. Thyroid gave her the general push she needed, and after six months on it, she began to menstruate again.

This doesn't mean that thyroid will make an older woman menstruate if she has completely stopped. But it certainly may help her general condition.

Dr. William Bickers agrees again. He thinks thyroid is so important in menopausal treatment he also uses it almost as a routine. He finds, too, that very small doses are all that are needed.

Tranquilizers

By now you've discovered that this menopause business isn't exactly simple. Estrogen. Androgen. Thyroid. There are so many things your doctor may want to try.

Well, it isn't simple. And there *are* a lot of things.

Tranquilizers are one.

In certain cases, where tests show that no hormones are indicated, doctors find tranquilizers just enough to keep their patients comfortable and help them over the hump.

The story of Theresa Root is the story of a woman who went through her changing years with nothing but mild sedatives to help her. Theresa is a Hollywood literary agent, black-haired, vivacious, definitely the high-strung type. And literary agenting is high-strung work. It demands a full day at an office, constant negotiations, frequent cross-country trips. Yet in spite of the fact that Theresa had a really hard time of it—great spells of weakness and a curious sudden fear of crowds so great she was sometimes afraid to cross the street alone—in spite of all this, she got along on nothing but tranquilizers.

True, there were times during the day when she felt she couldn't take another minute. Then she obeyed instructions to lock the office door, take the receiver off the hook, lie down and take a ten-minute complete rest. This enabled her to be up and at it again.

Equally important, her doctor insisted she must never let a day go by *without* going to the office. "No matter how bad you feel, you must never get it into your head you can't work!" he said firmly. "Or can't cross the street. Or can't handle your job. Because to think that would be the worst thing that could possibly happen to you. Rest when you have to, but by all means keep on."

Theresa had a long menopausal pull. In fact, she was one of the rare cases where the change took many years. But tranquilizers, plus courage, plus the knowledge that her distress, though long, was temporary, saw her through.

(An extra word on this: Since tranquilizers can be addicting, they should be taken only as prescribed, and for as limited a time as possible. No woman should of her own accord continue to take them after the need for them has passed.)

ADDING TO THE ESTROGEN STORY

Estrogen favors the laying down of calcium in the bones. When a true deficiency of estrogen develops, the calcium is pulled out of an older woman's bones, especially the bones of her spine. As a result, her bones become lighter and more porous, and a condition called osteoporosis (literally "porous bones") develops. And as the bones in her spine become lighter and more porous, the spaces between them become smaller too, so that she shrinks in height. (I shrunk from four foot ten to four foot nine and one half. Imagine that!) Or the lighter bones at the top of the spine may cause the head to jut forward, forming a hump on the back called a "dowager's hump." Worse yet, the lighter bones at the bottom of the spine may cause the hipbones to become weaker, so that a woman breaks her hip and falls.

For actually, says New York's orthopedic surgeon Dr. Howard Rosen, an older woman doesn't fall and then break her hip, as most people believe. Her hip joint becomes brittle and her bone breaks, and then she falls. And this hip break happens about eight times as frequently in women as in men, probably due to progressive estrogen loss.

So, to repeat, estrogen is important as a possible preventive of osteoporosis and equally important are exercise and diet. According to some research, it is important to get calcium into your body by drinking three glasses of milk a day, or taking milk in the form of yogurt or cottage cheese. Other research stresses eating more vegetable proteins and less meat.

Dr. S. Georgeanna Jones is one doctor who prescribes estrogen for osteoporosis. She does so because she believes it stops calcium loss, at least temporarily. But when she does prescribe estrogen, she insists that her patients stop smoking, since smoking causes lung changes that interfere with calcium metabolism. And while she gives the estrogen only for a short time, she says that drinking milk or taking calcium gluconate tablets, plus stopping smoking, must go on forever.

Yet this is most important to remember: Estrogen pills are not "pills to keep you young." Nor pills that will "keep you feminine forever." There is no substance in the world that will keep you in a state of constant youth, as some far-out fads have promised to do. In fact, falling for far-out fads will only leave you sad and disappointed when you find that the miracles they so glibly predicted just didn't come off.

And taking estrogen pills as early as, say, age thirty-five, won't make you "skip the menopause." If anything, such treatment may do just the opposite—make your menopause more severe when it does come. For at age thirty-five, in all probability you will still be menstruating regularly, and regular menstruation proves you have plenty of your own estrogen. So taking more will do nothing for you; your body will just throw it off as waste. Worse, the extra amount may hurt you before it is thrown off. Since your hormone system works on that basic stop-and-go arrangement, too much estrogen taken in any form may only succeed in overloading your pituitary with "stop" signals, overloading it to the point where it does not send out its normal number of "go" signals to your ovaries. Your ovaries may then become so lazied up they stop working long before they should, and as a result you may end up with fewer sex hormones rather than more!

For these reasons, sober and sensible doctors like Dr. Robert Hall of the Columbia Presbyterian Hospital in New York says he seldom gives hormones to any woman under the age of fifty, or to any woman whose menstrual periods have not stopped for a full six months. And even after the age of fifty, or whenever it is your menstrual periods do stop, no sober and sensible doctor will give you any kind of hormone pills unless you have a real need for them. Happily, I must repeat again and again, about sixty to seventy percent of all women never show such a need. Their hormones dwindle so slowly they are protected by them practically to the end of their days. Or their adrenals secrete enough extra hormones to offset their natural loss.

There's every chance you may fall into this fortunate group. Most of my friends have. Though well into or past their fifties, Eve recently opened the first fine-art gallery in Long Island's Five Towns area; Dolly is a top-flight New York interior decorator; Olga lectures at the New School for Social Research; and Augusta is trying to develop new strains of African violets, meanwhile keeping her dentist-husband's waiting room full of exquisite experimental blooms. Yet none of these women has taken a single hormone pill. They have taken something else, however. They have adopted the positive philosophy of "Yes, I can!" and when they have felt full of the stress none of us escapes, they have countered it with, "Get up off your backside, and stop feeling sorry for yourself. Move!"

And if they should ever get to the point where they do need hormones, none of them says she wants them to the point where they create artificial menstrual periods, something that also was popular for a while. Practically all of the hundreds of women I have questioned agree it is ridiculous to create artificial menstrual periods in one's fifties, sixties, or seventies for any reason. In fact, they say they are delighted to be rid of them, especially since they can get most of the other hormone benefits they may need without bothering with *that*.

What Hormones Can and Cannot Do

When I say "other hormone benefits" let me for emphasis repeat what they are, so you will be sure what hormones can and cannot do: Hormones taken after the menopause can help to prevent osteoporosis with its accompanying shrinkage of height and broken hips. They can possibly prevent or cut down the incidence of coronary attacks. They can increase resistance to physical and mental fatigue. And they can almost certainly relieve a dry, itching, or shrunken vagina that makes sexual relations far less pleasant than they were meant to be.

But here's what they cannot do, or do in such a small way it hardly counts:

They cannot cure osteoporosis or a broken hip once you have them.

They cannot stop your face from wrinkling or, if it has already wrinkled, make it smooth again. The reason for this is that your vagina has been a prime target for estrogen all your life; your face not nearly as much. Stop and think: don't most women's faces get older-looking and develop some wrinkles between the ages of thirty and fifty when they still have a rich quota of estrogens? If hormones can stop this, why don't they do it then?

Besides, the older one gets, the more resistant one gets to the restorative effect of any medication. A young person is like a budding plant that quickly perks up when treated with fertilizer. A full-blown plant responds more slowly, until there comes a point where fertilizer has little effect.

To be sure, some women just happen to inherit a tendency toward a smooth, unlined face that lasts almost indefinitely. Other women don't. One woman who dashed off a book on "pills to keep you young" had to admit later that most of her so-called rejuvenation was due to the fact she'd recently had her face lifted by plastic surgery.

Something all older women can do to help their skins is to use a moisturizer. Another is to avoid the sun like the plague. Or if they feel they have to sun themselves, use a sunscreen lotion containing PABA. PABA is a natural ingredient of the body contained in things like urine and sweat. Made in the laboratory as a chemical to be used as a sunscreen ingredient, it absorbs much of the strong ultraviolet light that would otherwise be absorbed into the skin. So read the label before you buy a lotion, or ask your druggist to give you one containing PABA.

Dr. Norman Orentreich, an authority on aging skin, explains why women have to be especially careful to avoid sunburn. In the October 1979 issue of *The Reader's Digest* he says: "All my laboratory research suggests that female skin ages faster than male skin because estrogen thins the skin." And thin skin, alas, while soft and pretty, is more susceptible to lines and wrinkles than thick skin. So if you are outdoors a lot, even in the winter when the sun can also be bright, use a moisturizer, and skip face creams that contain estrogen, and lotions that don't contain PABA. Best of all, keep your face out of the sun as much as possible because the sun can do as much if not more harm than good.

Not Retard Aging

Not only is there no known medication that can retard wrinkling, there is no known medicine that can retard aging in general.

In his book *The Ageless Woman,* Dr. Sherwin C. Kaufman talks about the Swiss doctor Paul Neihaus who claims to give a revitalizing treatment which he calls "cellular therapy." After treatment he gives each patient a document which says she has received several injections of "fresh cells of hypothalamus, placenta, marrow bone, kidneys, thyroid, parathyroid, heart, arteries, ovaries, and adrenals." This rather strange combination, Neihaus adds, "will keep her young and prolong her life."

One woman in her fifties paid many thousands of dollars for these injections, says Dr. Kaufman. Yet only a year after she received them she began to have severe hot flushes and night sweats just like some of her friends did. When she wrote a surprised letter to the Swiss doctor he replied, "Your unpleasant symptoms will disappear within three months." They did not. His expensive treatment had been worthless though her check had been good.

The writer W. Somerset Maugham regularly had these injections too, and swore they helped him live to the age of ninety-one. Maybe. But did you ever see pictures of Maugham as he aged? He became as wrinkled as a prune.

To repeat still again:

Take estrogen only as ordered by your doctor, and only in the way he or she prescribes.

Don't sample a few of your friends' pills to see if they will be helpful.

Don't lend your pills to a friend to try.

Don't step up the dose on your own inspiration. If one pill a day makes you feel well, don't think that two will make you feel better. They won't.

Remember that estrogen is powerful medicine. A small amount may prove a kind friend. A large amount an enemy.

Always the general rule is: take the smallest amount of estrogen for the least possible time, preferably with breaks between. Also expect slow results. Claudia, who started a difficult menopause at age fifty, took a very small amount, stopped as her doctor had suggested when most of her symptoms disappeared, then started again if and when they reappeared. Each time she started again she reported to me gaily over the phone: "My pills are working again! I sleep through the night. I'm full of energy. And I remember things I had forgotten. It is as if my life were like a tape recorder running itself backward. Wowee!"

Now she has stopped entirely, and at age fifty-two is working like a beaver at a successful book-distributing business she started in her own home.

SUMMING UP

So to sum up this important chapter:

The menopause is not the only change you've gone through. It is merely one of the long series of changes you've been going through ever since you were born.

And during this particular change it may be normal and natural for you to have no trouble at all. On the other hand, it may be equally normal and natural for you to be physically swept as by lightning, and to suffer many temporary discomforts and pains.

Your doctor can help you lessen these discomforts and pains. If you are troubled in any way, swallow any false modesty you may have and go straight to a good up-to-date physician. He has medicines at his command of which the old-timers never dreamed, and is getting new ones every day.

But do not overdo even the best medicines. Remember that, whatever happens, time and nature are on your side. There will be spontaneous improvement in a few months, or at most, a few years. I say years because all great changes take place more slowly in an older woman than in an adolescent girl.

In the words of Walter Cannon: "As far back as the dawn of history the fathers of medicine recognized that repair takes place after injury, health after pain, and though much of this self-repair takes time, the healing forces will restore you to health and efficiency if only you give them the chance which time alone provides."

So give yourself the benefit of treatment if you need it. But also give yourself the benefit of time. Take treatment carefully, and add to it optimism and hope. Do not expect it to "turn time backward and make you young again." Do expect it to help you move as smoothly as possible into the good years to come.

8

How You Can Help Yourself

Once when I was recovering from a serious illness and making little progress my family doctor rather impatiently said to me: "If only I could cut your head off, I would have you well in no time."

What he meant was, if only he could stop me from thinking negative thoughts. If only he could put a lock on my brain and treat my body without my mind butting in.

During the menopause positive thoughts are vastly important. Indeed, they're so important that there's no time in your life when you'll need positive thoughts more than you do now. This is because perhaps at no other time since you were born have so many upsetting things been happening to you at once.

Nature has, by coincidence, so planned it that just when you are physically swept by lightning, emotional shocks occur as well. Your children come of age and get ready to leave you. Your husband goes through his own mid-life crisis. Your parents start to get their own age or financial complications and reverse the role you have become accustomed to; possibly becoming dependent on you as you were once dependent on them.

And these things can happen to a woman when she feels least able to cope with them, or at least doesn't *want* to cope with them. Who wants to rearrange the home in which she has been living for years? Who wants to endure her children leaving her, though leave her they must?

So the hot flashes, the anxiety, the fatigue, the insomnia can stem from many causes. Upsets of body can be joined by upsets of mind.

But for the mind-upsets there is hardly a chance in a thousand you'll need a doctor. Here you can definitely help yourself. As psychiatrists constantly remind us, the human mind is capable of enormous powers of self-help. The same mind that helped bring about an illness can help bring about its cure.

So let's take the various discomforts in turn, and see what your mind can do to relieve them regardless of any medicine you may take.

HOT FLUSHES OR FLASHES

The best thing you can do for the flashes is to stop worrying that they will do you some permanent harm. Realize that they are not "weakening," but are a nuisance at worst.

You may have been unduly worried about this because many people connect perspiration with weakness. This is because perspiration usually accompanies a high fever, and so has become associated in our minds with something bad.

But what we forget is that it is the fever and the poisons causing the fever which are weakening us, not the perspiration. The perspiration is incidental. In fact, without a fever, perspiration is often beneficial. Don't we pay for the privilege of working up a good perspiration in a whirlpool or Turkish bath? Or in a "reducing cabinet" that makes us sweat and lose water until we take a drink and get the water back? And we certainly perspire when we jog, play tennis, take a brisk walk, or engage in any other healthy exercise.

No, perspiration isn't bad in itself by any means. The flushes may be supremely uncomfortable at times, but they are no worse than that.

INSOMNIA

You can also greatly help the insomnia by realizing that this, too, is not "weakening." That lack of eight hours' sleep every night cannot "drive you out of your mind."

Certainly it is not pleasant to lie in bed and toss and long for sleep that does not come. But you will be helped if you will remember that in the long run most of us get as much sleep as we need, just as we get as much food as we need. Parents used to worry their heads off when a child didn't want to eat. Now we know enough to let him be; tomorrow, of his own accord, he may make up for it and eat so much he doesn't seem to know when to stop. It's the same way with sleep. You can't sleep at night? Let it pass. Toward morning you may drop off so soundly you can hardly wake up.

I remember a distinguished navy captain who had charge of a convoy of ships going back and forth to England during World War II. He was well in his fifties at the time and he told me about a devastating week he put in at the height of the submarine menace since there were eighty ships in that particular convoy, all carrying precious cargo. For seven days and seven nights he never took his clothes off, or left the bridge. The most he could do was to snatch a few minutes rest sitting up in full uniform in a chair.

Naturally, when at last he reached shore, he was ready to drop. He was sure he needed sleep for another week at least. But he got in barely ten hours when the call came to turn around and take a new convoy out again! And he had no choice but to obey.

It is years since he told me the story. And life still owes him that missed sleep, for he never did get it. But did it hurt him? Not in the least.

I don't mean that we could all do as the captain did. But keep in mind that loss of sleep has never permanently hurt anyone, especially if the loss comes from such a normal thing as the menopause or the passing of the years.

Maybe the best remedy for sleeplessness I ever heard was given me by a woman I met in a restaurant in New York. I was having lunch alone one noon when a fine-looking white-haired woman sat down beside me. I was attracted by her bright scarf, and even more by her bright face. Here was a woman, I thought, who surely looked ageless and vital and warm. Yet when we got to chatting she told me she, too, was going through the menopause and insomnia was her particular problem. However, she thought she had it licked. "I always leave some little job, like tidying up a bookcase, undone at the end of the day," she told me. "Purposely undone. Then if I can't sleep at night, I simply get up and finish the job. The next day I'll also leave something undone. The motion of my hands takes the overexcited blood away from my brain, and pretty soon I go back to bed and doze off. It always seems to work." I personally say poetry to myself. Or sing old songs. Or relive a fond memory. Each of us can develop our own tricks.

Leave something undone for your hands to do! I don't think I've ever heard of a saner way of beating insomnia, or indeed a better philosophy of life. If you add to that the realization that no possible lasting harm can come to you if you don't sleep for a few hours, then you, too, should have the problem licked.

ANXIETY

Anxiety is another villain that often plagues our changing years. It isn't always a specific kind of anxiety either—the kind that you can lay your finger on. It is rather a general anxiety—the kind that makes you feel just vaguely anxious over everything—your children, your husband, your future, the whole wide world. And sometimes it can be so bad you may have regular "anxiety attacks," since the older you get the more vulnerable you become to fears and negative emotions of all kinds. If this happens, you can go into a real whirl.

I had such a general anxiety-attack during my menopause. My husband and I had recently bought a farm, an old stone house in the country such as I had always dreamed of. We bought it primarily as a summer home, but we also hoped to learn enough to farm it; make it pay its way with a few cows we would milk and tend ourselves.

This had been a dream of ours for years, but now that it was a reality I was suddenly petrified. We had just made the down payment and settled matters in the lawyer's office, and I was alone in the empty house trying to clean it up a bit before our furniture arrived. Unexpectedly it happened. An anxiety attack.

The kind of thing I had heard of but never experienced. An overwhelming attack of general worry and fear that had me floored.

Everything connected with the farm deal suddenly frightened the life out of me. The house frightened me; I was afraid of the low ceilings, the small windows, the very walls. The future frightened me: What did we city slickers know about farming? We'd lose our shirts, sure thing. The country frightened me. What made me ever think I liked the country? The country was a horrible place. How would we keep warm if we decided to stay the winter? Would we find household help? How would we meet the next payment? Two city people in our fifties. We were mad to set out on a venture like this.

My head whirled with any and every possible objection. If the one payment we had made hadn't been so substantial and flight had been possible, I would have flown from this strange, fearful house like a child from the dark.

An hour later, however, my furniture arrived. My heart still thumping, and trembling all over so badly I hardly knew what I did, I made myself unpack and arrange it as best I could. Then, worn out more from the mental struggle than the labor, I set about making myself some much-needed lunch on the big coal stove.

As I cooked, my eye happened to light on the coffeepot in my hand. "Why, that looks like my old coffeepot from home," I said to myself. And a second later: "Why, that *is* my old coffeepot!" Then I noticed the coffee mug in my hand. "Why, that's my old coffee mug too, and there's my old rocker. . . . And the bedspread my mother crocheted."

I know it sounds like a miracle, but from that moment most of my anxiety left me. Unwittingly I had done exactly the right thing—carried something known into an experience of the unknown. I had used the same instinctive wisdom that had made the ancient seafaring Greeks carry their household gods with them when they sailed to foreign shores. The simple act of holding my own coffee mug, making coffee in my own pot, had made this strange house into a familiar house. I wasn't afraid of it any more.

What's more, the anxiety never came back. We managed with cows, we managed with help, we managed somehow to make the place pay its way. None of my fears were realized.

I learned quite a lesson from that attack. I learned that most of our fears are mainly the fear of the unknown. We overrate security, especially as we get older. We are so sure security is the main answer to life that we blindly hold onto a known way of living even when it's bad. But if we somehow find the courage to push ahead and do the thing we're afraid of, then the new life may turn out to be better than the old.

Maybe that's what Jesus had in mind when He said: "Take no thought for the morrow." Maybe what He meant was, "have no anxiety about the morrow." Plan ahead, yes. But do not look ahead with apprehension. For once you are actually in the middle of doing something, it may turn out to be easier than you could possibly have guessed.

Another story told to me by a neighbor illustrates this point so beautifully I must tell it as well.

My neighbor knew a man who had a heavy, old-fashioned square piano he no longer wanted. He decided to give it to the Salvation Army. The legs were off; the keys were mostly gone; worse, it seemed to be locked and he had lost the key. But it was made of genuine rosewood and he thought the Army could at least sell it for the wood.

The Salvation Army people duly arrived, with two rather undersized men to do the moving job. Usually it takes at least two big men to lift a piano, and the donor was skeptical about these men making it to the street since he lived up several flights. But they appeared to lift it easily nonetheless and carry it down, the owner going along and shouting instructions as they rounded the curves in the stairs.

When they got out to the truck, however, the keyboard cover, probably from being shaken in the descent, flew open. When this happened one of the men exclaimed in surprise: "Why, it's a piano!" "So it is," the second man replied. "If I'd have known it was a piano I could never have lifted it." "No," said the first man. "Neither could I."

I have often thought of that story and it's punch line: "If I'd have known it was a piano I could never have lifted it." That's simply another way of saying: "Take no thought for the morrow." Is there a better way of warding off general anxiety than sometimes deciding *not* to think about what's ahead of us? Realizing we'll be able to summon all our forces and meet the challenge somehow, somewhere when it comes?

HEART PALPITATIONS

Another place you'll want to help yourself during this time, is in the matter of the heart palpitations—a tightening or pounding in the chest that can make you feel on occasion as if you're about to burst.

The best advice here is: after an EKG and a stress test prove that there's nothing wrong, pay no attention to them. I explained in the last chapter how in all probability they are not "heart trouble," or even anything remotely connected with it. Nine chances out of ten they are glandular in origin, and so, as the scale rights itself, and if you help by cutting down on caffeine, they will go quietly away.

In the meantime ignore them. Constant attention to *any* part of the body sends an extra supply of blood there, resulting in still more congestion and pain. The heart in particular acts this way.

Dr. Josephine A. Jackson explains why in her book *Outwitting Our Nerves:* "Man can live at the equator or exist at the poles. He can eat almost anything and everything, but he cannot stand long self-contemplation. The human mind can accomplish wonders in the way of work, but it is soon wrecked when directed into the channels of worry. In other words, hands off! Or, rather, minds off! The surest way to disarrange any function is to think about it. It is a stout heart that will not change its beat with a frequent finger on the pulse, and a hearty stomach that will not act up under attention. . . . Know enough about your body to counteract false suggestions; fulfill the common laws of hygiene . . . then forget all about the rest."

While Dr. T. A. Ross of London, England, put his advice this way: "People have often a quite impossible standard of health. They have created an ideal person who always has a perfectly comfortable body which never aches. They really do not seem to know that everyone has discomfort nearly every day. That pain can exist in a person who is in perfect health."

If you listen to these two wise physicians, if you realize you can have occasional pain and still be in perfect health, then you will be helping yourself a very great deal.

FATIGUE

Another problem you may encounter during the menopause is fatigue, a fatigue that can be a heavy burden indeed. For this weariness may bother you far more than insomnia, since insomnia comes only at night. It may be far more annoying than the palpitations or the flushes, since these come and go. But exhaustion can seem for the time being to stay on steadily for days on end.

There may be a physical cause for this fatigue—a temporary low supply of hormones. There may be an emotional cause, which is more subtle and harder to find. But if you know about it, you may decide your fatigue is *purely* emotional. In that case hormones won't help it at all.

The idea that fatigue can be emotional is quite new. It stems from our modern knowledge of psychology. Research men, especially those who worked with soldiers during the two world wars, found, to their surprise, that weariness was largely tied up with three things—worry, boredom, and defeat.

Take an example. During World War I the English Army suffered a bad setback at Mons and had to retreat. This retreat was a frightful ordeal lasting a week. During that week the men marched day and night under constant enemy fire, never daring to stop to sleep and hardly to eat. At the end of this time they were in a state of complete exhaustion, and the army doctors figured that practically all would need long hospitalization because of battle fatigue. Yet after only a few days of rest many of these same men turned around and helped win the Battle of the Marne!

The doctors could only figure it this way: Without the challenge of the new battle the men might have stayed exhausted from their retreat indefinitely. But under its challenge, and with a possible victory ahead of them instead of defeat, they called upon their hidden emotional reserves and their fatigue became a thing of the past. They fought like fresh men.

If you stop and think about it, you, too, are in many ways like a soldier during your menopause. You, too, may be retreating from a battle—the battle of raising a family. You need new challenges so you can throw off your tiredness and carry on. Or business battles. Or the inevitable disagreements that come from living with the same person for many, many years.

MAKE A CHOICE

What can you do to change boredom into possible victory? First and foremost, you can get out of your home for at least part of the day. Get out and do challenging things.

You can for instance: go back to school under one of the new continuing-education plans and get a college, or college-equivalent degree. Here is part of a letter a woman sent to the Boston psychiatrist Dr. Jean Baker Miller: "I was in my kitchen for twenty-five years. Then I got a college-equivalent degree. I feel so wonderful now. I have to pinch myself to see if I'm real! And ready to go out into the real world!"

Actually, there's nothing more real than helping children to grow, which the writer, along with her cooking and scrubbing, had been doing those twenty-five years. Yet she hadn't felt "real" until now, when, as she said, she was ready to go out into the "real world."

What is the "real world?" In her book *Toward A New Psychology of Women,* Dr. Miller says it is a place whose activity affects you—you pay its predetermined taxes, buy its food at the price it sets, drive according to its speed laws—but somehow you do not believe you affect it. Unless you have been active politically or part of some important social movement, you feel you have no influence on it. But once you get outside, you *know* you have some influence. And it is this knowledge which adds to your sense of fulfillment. Also, it's extremely fulfilling to get control of your life by even a boring job that puts bread on the table and shoes on your feet.

Being Fulfilled or Liked

Yet there's a catch here. Some women aren't sure they want to become fulfilled. They're afraid that if they do, they won't be liked. Men in particular won't like them. Some men will get so hysterical they'll call them "bitches," "man-eaters," or even "castrators," and leave them severely alone.

And this worries women, especially older women whose training has been different from that of boys. From childhood on they have seen boys urged to beat other boys, to become stronger, smarter, do anything to get ahead. While girls in main have been told to become pretty, well-mannered, be only mildly competitive for fear that otherwise they will be "left on the shelf."

Who has been behind this kind of teaching? Frightened men. Socrates knew this thousands of years ago. That wise Greek said, "Let women become equal and they will become superior." And because they deeply knew that women would become superior they held them down; treated them as a subordinate group. Told them they were too weak, too delicate, too emotional, too incompetent to try to do anything more difficult than be pleasing and polite.

Yet when during World War II these "weak" and "incompetent" women were called upon to do the kind of hard factory work that freed men for combat, the same men who had insisted they couldn't possibly succeed at it had to admit they had succeeded very well. But they hedged on the statement, and praised women for women "manning" the factories, though it still might be a better idea, they said, for women to go back home and learn how to bake better bread.

A Long Time

It has taken women a long time to dare once more to break out of their shells. To prove they can become jockeys, film directors, commercial pilots—do all the things they were too "dumb to do."

I'm sure Ellie Smeal did a great deal of soul-searching before she was able to break out of her role as housewife and become the president of the National Organization of Women. Perhaps even Mary Martin, who came out of retirement at sixty-three to return to Broadway, had her doubts. (I saw Mary Martin in a TV interview holding nervously onto Ethel Merman's hand, while Merman was assuring her she could succeed.)

Has this stopped men from liking Ellie Smeal, Mary Martin, and other highly successful women? Maybe a little. Possibly these women are lonely as a result, but if you ask them they'll tell you it's worth it. Some loneliness is the trade-off we all have to make in order to get to and stay on the top.

Small Jobs Versus Big

We can't all, to be sure, get to the top. But we can get out and work at smaller jobs. Jobs that will earn our own and others' respect.

Granted it's hard to start or restart at maturity. Alright, we'll still have to do it. And we can by getting over our feelings of inadequacy, and concentrating on our strengths instead.

Take the New York City woman who had been a nurse's aide in her twenties but was curtly refused a similar job in her fifties. What did she do? Knowing she had been a *good* nurse's aide who was merely a little stale, she went back to nursing school, studied up on all the new ways, and within a few months after graduation had a job in the "real world" as a regular nurse at Goldwater Hospital. And she enjoyed it so much that when she came to the mandatory retirement age of seventy she lied about her age and told them she was only fifty-eight. And the hospital directors enjoyed *her* so much they winked at her deception and let her stay on for twelve more years, until she was eighty-two.

Then take the meter maid in Northampton, Massachusetts. She hadn't worked for years either, and when she heard that meter maids were wanted, she was so scared she walked by the application place three times before she summoned up the strength to go in. Certainly she's now out all day in all weathers, but she feels she's doing a necessary service in the "real world" by handing out parking tickets, because if she didn't the cars on Main Street would never move on.

SOME PRACTICAL TIPS

As usual, I'd like to give a few practical tips. If you're looking for a job in an office it helps greatly to prepare a written résumé of your work experience. The tip here is to write the résumé backward.

List a college degree first, if you have one, because then it will be taken for granted that you have a high school certificate. The same with all the jobs you held in the past; list the last one first. Also when you describe those jobs, stress the positive things you did while holding them. Say things like "I organized this" or "I initiated that."

Also keep your résumé short, preferably on one page. And when you've finished show it to a few businesspeople you know and ask them, "If you were hiring someone, would this résumé impress you?" If they say it wouldn't, revise it until they say yes.

Volunteer Work

Volunteer work used to be looked down upon. No longer. Especially if it is the kind of volunteer work that gives you self-confidence and helps you acquire skills. It takes skill to be a successful club president or community fund-raiser. To organize a hospital library and select the kind of books patients will want to read. So don't minimize things like that in your résumé either.

Most important, volunteer work gives you that indispensable item of self-esteem. If you volunteer for a rape hotline and accompany a rape victim to a police station and speak up for her when she's too distraught to speak up for herself, she'll be extremely grateful, and your self-esteem will go up when she tells you so. If you sing well in a church choir, it will go up when the congregation tells you so, too.

Create Your Own

And if you can't sing well, create your own job, be like Gretchen Grant, a former actress, who thought up and launched frozen piecrust. Or Charlotte Cramer, who was the originator of prepared cake mixes. Or Lydia Pinkham, who had to concoct her famous patent medicine for years in the basement of her Boston home before it caught on.

Or the Texas woman who reads stories over the telephone to shut-in children. Or the Malden, Massachusetts, woman who supplies nearby hotels with cut flowers for their tables. Or the New York woman who caters weddings and parties, and swears she can supply everything at twenty-four hours' notice except a bride. . . .

I could go on and on.

Do you have to be particularly clever to think up money-making ideas like these? No. Or particularly artistic? No. Just persistent. Persistent and courageous enough to overcome your natural fears and inertia and make the start. To tease and goad yourself into getting out of your rut.

And how do you find out what to make a start at? That's not as difficult as you may think. You can take aptitude tests in almost any large city. You can also do something at home. You can sit down and think back to the days of your youth. What did you like to do then? For the strange thing is, what you *like* to do is usually what you *can* do or learn to do. At least you'll be so happy at it that it's far better than making more money at something else. Is it sewing? Then something connected with sewing is your answer; running an alteration shop is just one idea out of hundreds since many dressmakers hesitate to take on alterations so there's always a place for a woman who will. Is it working with people? Then something connected with "service" is your answer. Opening a private kindergarten. Even a special kind of baby-sitting service. There's an organization in New York that calls itself *Grandmothers Incorporated;* its expert baby-sitting services are in constant demand.

Or is it cooking? Then working with food is the thing for you. There seems to be absolutely no limit to the amount of good homemade food people will buy. Not only cakes and candies but sauces, jams, herbs, fancy sandwiches. I had lunch recently with a woman who boasts she "put herring on Park Avenue." She wasn't exaggerating. She did.

So take a deep breath; straighten your hair the way a man straightens his necktie; beg or borrow a small amount of capital, and plunge. For the nth time, it won't be easy. But then, is playing contract bridge easy? Or doing crossword puzzles? Or any of the other things you may be doing now? And anyway, with the most precious thing in the world, your ego, at stake, it's worth the effort. No matter if it's as hard as getting six teeth pulled, think of the flutter you'll cause with your family when you casually mention at the dinner table that you've made your first profit in the competitive business world.

Active, Not Passive, Hobbies

But suppose you don't want or need a job, and are looking for a hobby instead. Then by all means make it a purposeful and valuable hobby. Valuable to you and to the community. Also one with a forfeit attached.

By forfeit I mean one where you suffer some loss if you don't keep up with it—suffer in some tangible way. For the trouble with most hobbies is that they have no forfeit connected with them. You start, say, doing watercolors at home with a great spurt of energy on Monday. You don't feel so well, so you vacillate about it on Tuesday. Wednesday there's a good movie playing up the street, so you skip it altogether. And Thursday you drop it for good. But if you've signed up for a course in watercolors and paid a nonrefundable fee in advance, then you'll jolly well keep at it no matter what the distractions. It's what my mother used to call "paying the policeman." I've tried it. It works.

And certainly you'll want to make it an active hobby rather than a passive one. A passive hobby means sitting still and listening to concerts or lectures. Women are always hoping that doing this will somehow bring them peace. But it won't. Concerts and lectures are fine *after* a day of creativity. But there's a hundred times more self-esteem to be gained from one hour of struggling actively to learn to play a lowly instrument such as the harmonica, than by weeks of listening passively to Previn, Ozawa, and Bernstein combined.

Too Long a Rest May Have Drawbacks

But job or hobby or whatever, nothing could be worse now than a good long rest. The idea of a long rest is so tempting that, unless you hurry up and find a creative substitute, it's ten to one that you may settle for it.

The idea of the rest cure was invented by Dr. S. Weir Mitchell, a distinguished physician of his day. Dr. Mitchell acted on the theory that our nerves are something apart from the remainder of our bodies. A sick person had sick nerves which had to be made healthy by special "feeding" in the form of rest. So he ordered his patients into bed to get this needed feeding, and kept them there for indefinite periods of time. But he had his own twist. Instead of making his patients comfortable, Dr. Mitchell made them miserable. He denied them all visitors and would not let them do a thing, even read. More, he forbade them to talk about their symptoms to anyone, including a nurse. They were to do nothing but lie and stare at the ceiling, making themselves so unhappy they wouldn't malinger when he decided they were ready to get up.

Today we've forgotten the original plan of the rest cure and do just the opposite. We go to Florida or California where we swap symptoms with fellow-resters the live-long day. Or we go to an expensive sanitarium where the main topic of conversation is our symptoms. What else is there to talk about? we ask.

On top of this, modern science has found that the nerves are *not* a special part of the body. There is no such thing as a "sick nerve." The nerves of the worst neurotic are as healthy as yours or mine; it is merely their behavior that is at fault; they simply send wrong messages to the brain. And as if this weren't enough to disprove Dr. Mitchell's theory, we also have found that during a so-called rest cure most people don't rest at all! They use up such a large amount of energy thinking about themselves and feeling sorry for themselves that, unless they are too ill to think, they get out of bed just as tired as before. For true rest includes recreation, which means "re-creation." And re-creation means being born anew. And being born anew comes only from a new incentive, a new interest.

In short, true rest or re-creation for a woman who's been out of the labor market or tied to a house for ten or twenty-odd years comes mainly from a creative new hobby or a creative new job.

REST SOLVES NO PROBLEMS

If this wasn't enough, a long rest (we're not here, of course, discussing short rests of a few hours) never solves major problems anyhow. The same problems you had when you went to bed are with you when you get up.

Take the case of Mabel Withers of Bridgeport, Connecticut. Mabel in the course of a single year during her menopause took four separate rest cures in a sanitarium. Each time while she was there she felt fine. Each time she arrived home she promptly got a relapse and had to be sent back. At last her family doctor, puzzling over the situation, went to see her and asked her a straight question: "What is there at home you are afraid of, Mabel?" Taken off guard, she blurted out: "My mother-in-law. She moved in with us a while back, and I can't stand living with her." The doctor pressed the matter further. Was it unavoidable that her mother-in-law live there? Yes, for the present it was. Did it look as if she might even have to live there indefinitely? Yes, it did. "Well, then," said the doctor, "you can't keep on dodging the situation indefinitely. A hundred rest cures won't do you any good under the circumstances. I suggest you summon up your courage and face the matter out once and for all. Go home and get adjusted to it instead of running away from it, unless you prefer to be an invalid for life." From somewhere Mabel did find the courage. She went home—and stayed.

You, too, can somewhere find the courage to face your problems instead of running away from them. Courage to rebuild your ego through your own efforts. Courage to let your children depart and lead their own lives.

If you do both these things—let your children go quietly, turn to other interests—then you have every chance in the world of getting them back. Of once more winning their admiration. Of having them seek out the wisdom and help and advice of yours they really need, but which, in order to break the silver cord, they have for the moment thrust aside.

As the psychiatrist Dr. Helene Deutsch is able to promise us: "The 'lost children' who have emancipated themselves will in time return. But only if they have really succeeded in achieving freedom. Only if the mother has understood her children's aspirations to liberty and not abused the methods by which she tried to attach them to herself. Then she has the happy prospects of repossessing them. But she must lose them first in order to possess them again."

The Chinese have a double meaning for the word crisis. They say a crisis is both a danger and an opportunity.

The changing years are critical ones, surely. They can bring danger, true. But they can also bring opportunity. It is largely up to you to choose.

9

You Can Keep Your Sex Life

It is midnight and Deborah Miller lies on her bed tossing restlessly. Hours pass. The clock strikes three, four, five. Her husband breathes heavily and deeply. She leans over and gives him a gentle pat, but she does not sleep herself.

Deborah and Jim have been married a long time, and recently a skipped menstrual period has greatly upset her. She knows she is inevitably approaching the menopause, and this may mean it is coming soon. And lately she has thought about her changing time often, and as she has thought, she has feared. All the old fears have come trooping into her mind. Will she lose her figure? Considering she has grown children, it is not a bad figure. Will her appearance drastically change? She never has thought of herself as a particular beauty, but still, what looks she has she would like to keep. Most important, will she lose her sexual attractiveness? Will she suddenly wake up one day to find all of that part of her life in the past?

Because sex to Deborah, nudging fifty, is far more than a physical thing; it is an emotional need that pulses through her being. The pattern of a whole relationship, the assurance that in her small, intimate world she still "belongs."

She cannot bear the thought that this pattern may be broken. But men, she has heard, continue their virility way into their late years. What if her femininity, that now matches his virility, fails her? What if this beloved man who lies sleeping beside her no longer turns to her for the comfort and succor she still yearns to give? What if—horrible thought—he turns to someone else?

What if nature has actually decreed that men turn to someone else? What if most men are potent in their fifties, their sixties, and even beyond, while their wives lose their ability to keep up with them? What if this is the universal plan?

Flushes, heart palpitations, nervous tension—Deborah can suffer these discomforts calmly if need be. But suffer *this* calmly? No. This is a thought too terrible to take.

Well, she need not take it. Nor need you. For fear of losing your sexuality, like so many other fears, is quite unfounded in fact. It is a myth based on a whole series of ancient misconceptions—misconceptions that, like a child's bogeyman, vanish when you look them straight in the eye.

The first misconception comes from the idea that there is an exclusive connection between your sex organs and your sex feelings. Some of us have at some time had thoughts like this: "When I was a child I had few estrogen hormones and my ovaries were not sending out eggs. Therefore I had no sex feelings. It only stands to reason then that when my ovaries are no longer sending out eggs my sex feelings will depart too."

Perhaps you've bolstered up this line of thinking by recalling what you know about eunuchs. Eunuchs, you know, are men who have lost their testicles, and therefore most of their androgens, through an operation or accident. And, as a result, isn't it true they have no sex life?

Then you may recall something about animals. Don't castrated roosters and hens lose their sex lives completely when they lose their sex organs? Moreover, don't even ordinary animals lose their sex drive once they are no longer able to bear young? Some animals, you know, have certain periods of "heat" during which the male dog can scent the female dog a block away, and the stallion grazing in the pasture rears and whinnies as the mare comes down the road. But once these periods of heat are over, the male dog walks disdainfully by the female, and the stallion keeps on with his grazing without giving the mare a second glance.

Don't animals also prove: no active sex organs, no sex desire or charm?

And if this weren't enough to upset you, perhaps you've done a lot of thinking lately on the subject of religion. (Many women get a rebirth of religious feeling around the time of the menopause.) You may have said to yourself: Don't the great religions teach that sex exists mainly for the creation of children? So when the creation of children is no longer possible, doesn't sex activity become sinful? Or, at the very least, not nice?

SEX UNFOLDS SLOWLY

First, let's talk about the belief that you had no sex feelings before puberty. This is not true. Modern science has found that sex feelings are present even before birth. Very young children discover their sex organs and react to them with pleasure, like the three-year-old boy who had a spontaneous erection while his mother was drying him after his bath, and said, "Mommy, I feel good all over, but I feel best of all down *there*." And as to hormones, there are enough active sex hormones flowing through a child's body to be counted from the age of four on. It may be the presence of these hormones that cause almost all youngsters to masturbate for a time.

To no person on earth does sex suddenly arrive in full splendor at puberty. It developed gradually before that, and continues to develop for many years.

SEX DEPARTS SLOWLY

Yes, sexuality unfolds and comes to full splendor slowly. It climbs from birth to adolescence, reaches a plateau where it stays for many years, then descends even more slowly than it climbed. Did it take many years to develop? It will take many, many years after the menopause to decline, and in women sometimes it does not decline at all.

For now, after the menopause, there are other factors present besides hormones. Now hormones do not tell the whole sex story by a long shot. There are other factors present that are equally powerful. These are psychological factors, the factors of habit and memory, which in some ways are the most powerful of all.

THE PSYCHOLOGICAL FACTORS OF HABIT AND MEMORY

What do we mean by "the psychological factors of habit and memory?"

We mean that sex is a physical drive, one of the strongest we have. And because it is a drive, we don't have to learn how to make love. We do it at a certain time, just as a newborn baby reaches for the breast.

But sex is also a psychic or emotional drive. And because it is emotional, we enhance its pleasure by surrounding it with grace and beauty, just as we surround eating with grace and beauty. When he has a choice, no wise person bolts his food; he partakes of it at leisure on a clean cloth with gleaming silver and polished plates. He strives to transform the prosaic necessity of eating into a beautiful act.

The wise woman does the same with sex.

She enjoys it with her emotions as well as her body; enriches it with tenderness and love. She does not regard the sex act as a mere biological duty, something to have over and done with as soon as possible. Instead she builds up happy memories surrounding it; becomes a person who desires to repeat the experience, who, even after a temporary setback, wishes to carry on and lift lovemaking into one of the highest of human arts.

So hormones alone do not account for sexuality. Indeed, by the time a person reaches maturity, hormones play such a comparatively minor role that sex has been estimated to be due forty percent to pleasurable emotions, another forty percent to association with love and tenderness, and only twenty percent to hormones.

If emotional factors weren't so important, the stories I am about to tell you would be even more astonishing than they are.

STERILITY IS NOT
THE SAME AS IMPOTENCE

But before I can tell these stories I must sidetrack a little and talk more particularly about men to clear up a point that's often confusing. It is the difference between sterility and impotence.

Sterility is the inability to create children. Impotence is the inability to have an erection, or to perform the act of sex in the first place.

Impotence is thus a far more serious condition, when it comes to the pleasure of sex, than sterility. A man may be able to perform the sex act but still be sterile because he lacks sperm vigorous enough to beget a child, or because he has had a vasectomy and his sperm are blocked off.

Now obviously when, naturally or as the result of an operation, a man loses his sperm power, he does become sterile. But does he also become impotent? Does he lose all potency and pleasure? That is what most of us used to believe.

As a rule we were allowed to keep on believing it. Men who'd been castrated for medical or other reasons didn't make their private lives a subject of casual conversation. And slaves who'd been castrated for harem reasons—well, if the sultans thought such eunuchs were incapacitated completely, let them think!

Dr. Tauber's Pioneer Investigations

Some years ago Dr. Edward S. Tauber, of the Department of Psychiatry and Medicine of Columbia University, decided to conduct what was practically the first serious investigation on the subject.

First, he studied ancient literature. To his surprise he found that not only were castrated men known in primitive societies

centuries before Christ, but some of them were allegedly potent
or capable of sexual intercourse.

He next found that there were many eunuchs in ancient
Rome and Egypt. On some of them the operation had been performed after puberty, on some before, with differences in the results. If performed before puberty, the results were usually drastic: complete impotence was caused. But after puberty the
capacity for intercourse was sometimes spared. Roman literature
even told of a few harem-eunuchs secretly keeping harems of
their own.

Then Dr. Tauber searched further and found some modern
records. He discovered members of a Russian religious sect, the
Skopts, who were so overzealous they castrated themselves in
order to make sure they would lead an ascetic life. But one
member who had performed the operation on himself at the age
of twenty-one changed his mind later, returned to civil life and
married; notwithstanding the fact that he was now an absolute
eunuch by physical standards, he told of having daily intercourse
for the next twenty years.

Next Dr. Tauber found a barber who had been castrated by
the authorities as a habitual criminal in an Eastern country where
such things were still legal. Yet the barber had intercourse for
four more years. While still another man, a carpenter who had
been operated on at the age of twenty-five, told of losing all potency and desire for nine years, then regaining them when he fell
in love and married. In the carpenter's words, "The marriage was
entirely satisfactory sexually to both myself and my wife."

Finally Dr. Tauber quotes important, but little-known, modern research done by a German doctor, Dr. A. Lange. Dr. Lange
knew that most soldiers have always had the misconception you
may have had—that loss of their testes means total loss of their
potency. As a result, the wound most feared was a wound in the
sexual region. But after World War I Dr. Lange interviewed several hundred soldiers who had been wounded in this way. Fully a
third declared their fears had not been justified; potency had
remained. Some even admitted to a heightened activity and response.

Dr. Tauber now analyzed his findings and reached these conclusions:

First: Practically all the men who had preserved their potency had lost their testes after puberty, not before. For after puberty, there had been time for brain and nerve patterns to be built up; patterns far stronger than those built up in a child.

Second: Potency does not remain unless love and tenderness remain. In practically all the men studied, love and tenderness were strong elements in their lives.

Third: The most important single factor in successful sex is not the presence or absence of hormones. It is the presence or absence of fear of sexual failure. All the successful men were blessedly free of such fear.

Other researchers confirmed Dr. Tauber's work. They found that the later in life a man loses his testicles, the less drastic the result.

If boys, for instance, are castrated in childhood (a practice which used to be common in Italy to preserve their voices as boy-sopranos in church choirs until an 1870 law forbade it) the effect is quite complete. If done in their twenties, the effect is less; in their thirties much less, and so on down the line.

The researchers also found that the adrenals are the source of extra androgens in both men and women. In men, too, when the androgens from the sex organs dwindle, some androgens from the adrenals move in and take their place.

All this seemed to add up to proof positive: mature men, aided by the androgens from their adrenals, plus memory and habit patterns, and the presence of tender love, can continue to enjoy sex though their testes are no longer producing androgens.

What About Women?

But what about women? Eunuchs are, after all, extreme cases, and it's normal women we are concerned about here. In normal women does the same thing hold true?

Let's take the physical reasons first. Let's go back for a minute to the important difference between impotence and sterility.

A woman, like a man, can be sterile. She can be unable to conceive throughout her adult life because her ovaries, or some other reproductive organ, are for some reason not functioning properly. She also surely becomes sterile once her menopause is past.

But, unlike a man, a woman cannot be impotent, because potency demands active cooperation from a man. He either can perform the act of sex or he can't. But a woman's part in the sex-act is mainly receptive (which does *not* mean passive). And she can be receptive even though she does not enjoy what she is doing. When she does not enjoy sex, nonorgasmic is the word that doctors use.

The crux of the matter then becomes this: When a woman loses her ovarian hormones gradually during a normal menopause, or suddenly as the result of an operation, does she automatically become nonorgasmic? Does she stop getting pleasure from the physical side of love?

To try to answer this question, Dr. E. A. Gaston also did some research. Again he looked for extremes to prove his case—women with one or both ovaries surgically removed. He questioned sixty-five mature women about their continued enjoyment of sexual response under these circumstances. His findings were about the same as in the case of men: Fifty-three out of the sixty-five women reported either no change in their feelings, only a slight decrease in their feelings, or actual improvement.

Once more it looked as if the psychic factors of habit and memory far outweighed the physical loss.

WOMEN HAVE STILL ANOTHER ADVANTAGE

But ovaries present or ovaries absent, women have still another advantage over men when it comes to the enjoyment of sex.

This is the fact that they feel pleasure in more places.

Men enjoy sex mainly through one organ, the penis. Women

enjoy it through the vagina, but in addition it pulses through their breasts and tingles through the skin of their entire bodies. Especially it vibrates through the clitoris, the highly sensitive little organ located above the entrance to the vagina.

Dr. Alfred C. Kinsey pointed out that the clitoris is such a vital seat of sex pleasure that it may be even more important than the vagina. This is because the vagina is largely lacking in nerves, while the clitoris is not. As a result, a woman enjoys sex more through the clitoris than any other organ, so that even a woman who has undergone total hysterectomy can still enjoy the act of love. For such a woman still has her clitoris very much intact.

Here is what Dr. Kinsey says on this point in his chapter on intercourse in his book *Sexual Behavior in the Human Male:*

"The most common error which the male makes concerning female sexuality is the assumption that stimulation of the interior of the vagina is necessary to bring maximum satisfaction to the female. This is obviously based on the fact that vaginal insertion of the penis during coitus may result in orgasm for the female. It is a considerable question, however, how significant the stimulation of the interior of the vagina may be. It is certain that most of the physical stimulation which the female receives from actual coitus comes from the contact of the external areas of the vulva, of the areas immediately inside the outer edge of the labia, and of the clitoris, with the pubic area of the male during genital union."

If, then, even a woman who has had a complete hysterectomy can often enjoy the sexual act the same as before, how much better off is a woman going through a normal menopause! A normal woman still has everything intact—ovaries, cervix, vagina, *and* clitoris. These make her very rich indeed.

The net result is, to use the words of Dr. Robert N. Rutherford of Seattle, Washington: "Femininity surely does not end at the menopause. It lasts until seventy, and in some cases well beyond."

Or to quote the well-known story about the Princess Metternich. When someone asked the princess at what age a woman loses interest in sex, that lady is said to have quickly replied:

"You must ask someone else; I wouldn't know. You see, I am only sixty years old!"

MAYBE LESS VITALITY DURING THE ACTUAL CHANGE

There's no denying that during the actual changing years so many new and delicate internal adjustments may be taking place that your general vitality will be low. As a result, you may lose some of your interest in sex. And when you lose interest, you may not produce enough vaginal secretions to lubricate your vagina and make sex enjoyable.

But you can use a little jelly to help a dry vagina. A particularly good one is KY lubricating jelly, which is odorless, nongreasy, and used by surgeons to sterilize their hands. A particularly poor lubricator is Vaseline, which is not only greasy, but nonsterile.

Most important, you can be assured that when your interest in sex returns, many of your own secretions may return. No lubrication may then be necessary.

DIFFERENT IN DIFFERENT WOMEN

Moreover, as I said, loss of interest in sex does not occur in all menopausal women. Some find their enjoyment actually increased, if only because they no longer fear unwanted pregnancies. And those who find it lessened can use faith to replace lowered vitality. For faith in the future, plus a remembrance of good things past, keeps habits and nerve patterns unbroken.

If your interest in sex does temporarily depart, when it returns it may be at a lower and slower pace. But that, too, is natural. There is a different degree of keenness to all our appetites as time goes on. Many of us don't care to walk as far at fifty as we did at eighteen, nor to play as many rounds of golf. But that doesn't say we can't fully savor the walks we do take, the golf we do play, especially if we have kept in good physical condition. Many couples today enjoy the time after the menopause as a gentle second honeymoon. They are the ones who remember that sexual decline, like other declines, is extremely gradual, not fast and overwhelming as they may have feared.

If you have had a good sex life up to maturity, you and I and the manicurist down the block, and the saleswoman at the department store, and the housewife next door, and all the other millions of women everywhere, will no more wake up one morning and find sex-interest gone—just like that!—than you will wake up and find your hair has turned white in the night.

You Can, But Should You?

"But it's all very well for you to say sex enjoyment *can* continue in a mature woman," you argue back at me. "But *should* it continue? Equally important for my peace of mind is the answer to the question, 'Is it right and proper now?'

"Animals," you go on, "don't mate when they can no longer produce offspring. Aren't we supposed to be a higher order than they? . . . And what about religion? Especially religion? Don't many religions teach that sex without the possibility of conception is sinful? . . . And regardless of religion, doesn't tradition teach that it is simply not nice?"

These are apt questions. Vital questions. I shall answer them in turn. Let's start with animals.

Sex and Animals

Granted that female mammals have certain periods of "heat" or seasonal sex interest; granted they are uninterested when the seasons of heat are past. But what mammals do in the sex sphere no more holds good for humans than the fact that a cow lives on grass, or a horse on hay, makes grass and hay a fit diet for man.

The reason mammals mate only at certain periods of the year is a matter of survival. The first aim of any species is to keep its young alive, and in the mammal world this is a risky business.

If a wild colt, for instance, were to be born in a northern

forest during the winter months it might soon perish from the cold. So nature times the mating of its mother and father in such a way that the colt is born during the warm months only. This protects the colt and permits it to survive.

But this kind of timing isn't necessary among humans. We can wrap our babies in blankets and cradle them in houses no matter when they are born. So nature lets us conceive at any time of the year, though to this day there is still a mysterious upsurge of sex desire in the summer that results in an especially large crop of babies the following spring.

Then take the matter of the length of time of pregnancy. In a woman, pregnancy lasts nine months. In an elephant, twenty-five months. In some dogs, a mere six weeks.

Or take ovulation. A rabbit releases an egg from its ovary only during the stimulation of actual intercourse. In a rabbit, or a rat, too, for that matter, no intercourse, no egg.

But most women ovulate regardless of whether they have no intercourse or have it several times a week. Again the comparison does not hold.

No, it seems that we're not only a higher order than other mammals, we're an entirely different order. So the next time someone refers to sex as "the beast in you," show that you know better by holding your head high, and saying "sex is part of the God in you." It would be nearer the truth.

Sex and Religion

Now, as to the question of religion. Does religion consider sexual relations past maturity improper?

There are two major religions in our Western world—Christianity, which I will divide into the Protestant and Catholic followings, and Judaism. The only way to answer this is to examine the position of each.

Let's take first the Jewish religion, because its teaching on this matter is the simplest.

The Jews have never had a tradition of "mortification of the flesh." On the contrary, there has always been stress on marital unity, including the physical expression of love. Orthodox Jewish law went so far as deliberately to *tell* a husband to make love with his wife—even point out how and when he should do this at certain times of the month. For the Jews, therefore, sex between husband and wife has always been a ritual and a trust.

Next, Protestant teaching.

Protestant teaching has not been as clear-cut on the subject. Indeed, when I asked several leading Protestant ministers, a few answered that they had never thought of it. But not all of them answered this way. Bishop G. Bromley Oxnam, of the Methodist Church, New York area, said he had given it long and serious thought. Bishop Oxnam replied: "Protestants generally hold a very high and sacred opinion of sexual relations. There are some who seem to hold that sexual relations are justified solely for purposes of racial perpetuation. But Protestants see in sexual relations not only a sacred obligation to bear children, but also something of beauty to enhance the love of a man and a woman. The sexual ties are among the strong ties that bind the family, and when regarded as an expression of love they would, it seems to me, justify thoroughly the continuance of such relationships following the period when conception is no longer possible.

"In answer to your question, therefore, I speak in the affirmative. I believe the continuance of marital relations after conception is no longer possible, is not only proper but normal, beautiful, and sacred."

Dr. Leland Foster Wood, of the Commission of Marriage and the Home, Federal Council of Churches of Christ in America, had also given this subject much thought. He said:

"God Himself in His beneficent wisdom has made us with a strong attraction between the sexes. When this sexual attraction is used with understanding and mutual consideration in marriage, the sexual union becomes a symbol of a splendid dedication of a man and woman to each other and to their marriage.

"Their sense of oneness should grow and deepen with the years. It should enable them to face the middle and later years with high hope and confidence rather than anxiety or despair. Both for husbands and wives who fully understand the meaning of marriage and the interrelationships between the physical, emotional, and spiritual factors, the sex relationship after the menopause can still be a rich and rewarding expression of love, loyalty, and intimate oneness.

"The idea that the relationship of husband and wife must be radically changed at the time of menopause has neither religious nor scientific justification. The fact that the sex factor in some cases is a liability rather than an aid is one of the sad effects of poor sex education and of unnecessary fears. The Author of our being has designed the sex factor in marriage for the greater unity of husband and wife. 'They shall be one flesh, so they are no longer two, but one.'"

These Protestant statements speak for themselves.

Finally I tracked down the Catholic position.

Catholics teach that deliberate use of artificial birth-control methods is "against nature" and, so, sinful. They do not teach, however, that to have marital relations without using artificial methods is sinful. Nor is it sinful when pregnancy is unlikely to result.

Here is how this has been made clear.

Dr. Leo J. Latz, an eminent Chicago physician and himself a devout Catholic, was the first to become deeply stirred over the discovery of a new birth-control method called "the rhythm." It was called this because it was discovered that people could space their children by having relations at those times of the month when the woman's "rhythm" was against her conceiving. Since this did not involve the use of artificial methods, it was not "against nature," and hence received Catholic permission.

Dr. Latz proceeded to publish a book called *The Rhythm of Sterility and Fertility in Women,* which has run into many editions. He says in this book, quoting the Catholic scientist Cappellman, who in turn is quoting A. Ballerini, professor at the Catholic Gregorian University in Rome:

"Married people are at liberty, under mutual agreement, to observe perpetual abstinence; they are at liberty to observe continence for twenty or thirty years, and to postpone the consummation of their marriage up to a time when there will be no hope of procreating children; they are at liberty to make use of their marital rights even when the wife is certainly sterile and can no longer conceive because of her advanced years, provided the right is used in order to realize another purpose of marriage. . . ."

This "other purpose" is the celebration of a sacrament. Dr. Latz points out that St. Augustine taught "Marriage has a three-fold purpose—offspring, fidelity, the Sacrament." And St. Thomas states "The first end of marriage—offspring—belongs to man as an animal; the second—fidelity—as a human being; the third—sacrament—as a Christian.

"Nature does not direct marital intercourse among human beings as it directs copulation among animals," continues Dr. Latz. "It provides sex stimulation during the period of sterility as well as during that of fertility, and must be assumed to intend the marital act for other purposes than procreation. If the latter were Nature's only objective it could be taken care of by married couples uniting once about every fifteen months."

And Dr. Latz continued: "The procreation of children is not essential to marriage. Matrimony, in all its essentials, is had even though no children result from the union."

To my mind, the words which say that "married people are at liberty . . . to make use of their marital rights even when the wife is certainly sterile and can no longer conceive because of her advanced years" clearly indicate the time during and after the menopause. Sexual relations between married people before, during, and after the menopause therefore become permissible and in no way a sin.

But on such an important subject let's turn to an authority other than a Catholic doctor. Let's turn to the late Bishop Fulton J. Sheen's book *Peace of Soul*.

In his chapter called "Sex and the Love of God" Bishop Sheen says: "There is no more towering nonsense than to say that the Church is opposed to sex. She is no more opposed to sex as such than she is opposed to eating a dinner. Nature is not corrupt. Our instincts and our passions are God-given.

"The sex drive in man is at no moment an instinct alone. . . . Desire from its beginning is informed with spirit, and never is one experienced apart from the other. The psychic and the physical interplay.

"Our body is part of the universal order created and preserved by God. Love includes the flesh."

Let's climb still higher on the Catholic ladder.

Let's go up to the highest rung, to a quotation from Pope Pius XI. In 1936 Pope Pius issued an encyclical called *On Chaste and Christian Marriage*. In it he discusses the question: What is the official attitude of the Church toward continued sex between wife and husband when no children are likely to result?

On page 27 of the official English translation of this encyclical, as published by Sheed & Ward of London and New York, Pope Pius says: "Nor are those considered as acting against nature who use their [marital] rights in the proper manner, although on account of natural reasons either of time or of certain defects new life cannot be brought forth. For in matrimony as well as the use of matrimonial rights there are also secondary ends, such as mutual aid [and] the cultivating of mutual love."

The words "on account of natural reasons . . . of time . . . new life cannot be brought forth" clearly indicate the time during and after the menopause.

The teaching of the Church is still quite positive on the subject. Artificial birth control is condemned, but sex between married partners is praiseworthy, and a source of happiness and holiness even apart from the procreation of children. Of this there is no doubt.

Sex and the Sense of Shame

But church or no church, you still may not be convinced. Because for many of us there's still another kind of code—that of "what's being done." Bluntly you say: "But nice women don't *have* sex relations after a certain age. And when they do, they're ashamed of them. I knew a woman who had a so-called change baby who thought she'd die of shame. It was as if she shouted to the whole world: "I'm still indulging in sex!"

Well, the only thing to do about this sense of shame is to trot it out into the light with all the others. To ask, *Why* are some women ashamed? *Who* planted the shame? How did it start?

There are several theories.

Dr. Howard W. Haggard of Yale University says men planted it. In his fascinating book, *Devils, Drugs and Doctors,* he says men of olden times planted it in women so that they would consider childbearing their chief role in life, and feel guilty if they had sexual relations when they wouldn't, or couldn't, bear children. Dr. Haggard says men didn't do this maliciously; they did it to ensure the survival of the race.

In Biblical days the average length of a woman's life was no more than about twenty years, with the result that if she started childbearing at fifteen and lived to an average of twenty, that left her only five years in which to produce the next generation. She therefore had to be persuaded to produce fast and furiously, or the race would have died out. And when she was through producing, on the shelf she went. (Did you ever notice how many old men or patriarchs are mentioned in the Bible, but how few old women? That's because there weren't many old women. Because of lack of sanitary conditions, especially in childbirth, they just didn't live long.)

Then, in the Middle Ages, the urge for the fast production of children was even stronger, if possible. For during the Middle Ages the woman's situation was worse than before. As Dr. Haggard puts it: "The Middle Ages was the most unfortunate period in the history of womankind. Complete ignorance prevailed, without the skill of the early intuitive period or the knowledge of previous civilizations. . . . Womankind had indeed fallen on evil days."

The results in loss of life during childbirth were appalling. Dirty and unkempt midwives performed all deliveries, going from one childbed to another without bothering to wash their hands. Also, because of a crazy streak of religiosity, doctors, merely because they were men, were forbidden at the bedside. When a Dr. Werth of Hamburg in 1522 dared to attend a case of a woman in labor, he had to put on a woman's dress as a disguise. Even at that, he was discovered and burned at the stake. Add to this the constant epidemics like the Black Death during the Middle Ages, epidemics in which whole towns were swept away, is there any wonder that the few women who did manage to stay alive and healthy were prevailed upon to bear and bear? While the mortality was so high among babies that the only answer was to bear some more?

So we can't completely blame the men of earlier times if they stressed sex for conception mainly. Large families had to be the fashion, large enough to start with at least, so a few children could sneak through and survive. (My own grandmother was quite an ordinary example of her day. She bore seven children in seven years, starting at the age of sixteen. Two of them lived.)

But the situation today is different. Today, what with great strides in health and medicine, we are beginning to have more people in the world than we have room for. Look at the figures and judge for yourself.

The first reliable world census dates back to 1630. According to that census there were about four hundred million people in the world, after a very slow increase during all the previous centuries of recorded time. But then the spurt started. By 1830, or only two centuries later, the world population had almost doubled to eight hundred million. By 1900 it had doubled again to more than a billion and a half. By 1940 it was well over two billion; by 1950 more than two and a half billion. By 1978, the latest figures we have, to well over four billion. And it is still growing by leaps and bounds.

In other words, the number of people in the world has multiplied ten times since 1630. And students of population point out that if it keeps up at this rate it could double in the next twenty years. This would mean covering almost every available inch of the earth unless we stop the spurt and hold the population growth to zero. At this time in history, therefore, says Dr. Haggard, the older woman who can no longer have children deserves no censure but praise.

DR. LAWTON'S THEORY

The psychologist Dr. George Lawton has a different theory as to why older women have been taught to be ashamed to continue to ask for sex relations. In his book *Aging Successfully* he says that not men in general but men in *particular* planted this shame. Men who couldn't keep up with their women. Men who couldn't provide sexual enjoyment much longer, and so condemned it to save their manly pride.

Dr. Lawton states that some older men taper off in their potency between the ages of fifty-five and sixty. And since men between fifty-five and sixty usually have wives several years younger, what could be more natural than for these men to get it noised about that if their wives continued to ask for the pleasure they could no longer give it was definitely "not nice"?

In Dr. Lawton's words: "The menopause is seldom correctly understood. Menstruation ceases and a woman is no longer capable of bearing children. But there is no loss of sex desire or capacity; there may even be an increase . . .

"To say (therefore) that in every older woman there is a complete loss of sexual desire and capacity is a male fiction adopted secondhand by women."

Thus a few men have spread a false doctrine and made many women the victims of it. It's like the story of the fox and the sour grapes. The fox said, "If I can't have the grapes then you don't want them." So a few men have said, "If I can't have sex, then you don't want it." And women have swallowed this fiction whole.

The True Role of Sex at Maturity

What, then, is the true role of sex at maturity? How long can you look forward to keeping your sex desires, and how can you use them with beauty and dignity while they remain?

According to the best consensus of opinion, the answer is, to sixty, seventy, and beyond. As Dr. Earle Milliard Marsh, chief of the department of Gynecology of the Hazard, Kentucky, Regional Hospital, points out, "Sex in women can be continued after sixty, then up into the seventies and eighties! Women never grow old sexually; the men do a little, but very little. If a man or woman has a willing sexual partner, sexual activity continues with very little decline until old age."

Sex was given to you for far more than a physical purpose. It was given to you for a social and psychological purpose—so you can continue turning outward instead of inward. The experience of turning outward toward another person is the best way of keeping you turned outward toward the world.

Dr. Frederick Lund of Temple University expresses this well when he says in his book *Emotions of Men:* "Man could not be moved to any great ideal were it not for some need and longing within him—a need that turns him outside.

"We may sincerely doubt whether the tender emotions of love and affection, of sympathy, chivalry, and generosity would have evolved without the hormones and internal irritants provided by the prosaic sex glands.

"Nature made sex good; made it essentially wholesome and beautiful. . . . It is a communion of personalities . . . not mere physical attraction. It is the greatest outgoing force we have."

You as a woman need to exercise this outgoing force in the form of tender love all your life. You need especially to exercise it in your later years so you don't become "ornery" as some older people do—ornery because you turn all your emotions inward instead of out.

You also need sex so you can go on touching some other living thing to keep you physically and emotionally warm.

Sex and Warmth

The psychiatrists O. Spurgeon English and Gerald H. Pearson explain why we have this great need for touch: "It is important that married couples enjoy the sexual relationship for many reasons," they say. "In a culture making increasing demands on the individual for tolerance and patience and interest in things outside himself it is important that he be able to derive all physical and emotional satisfaction from marriage. The marriage relationship coming on at a time of increased social responsibility offers through the opportunity of a close physical relationship the chance to recapture some of the sustaining satisfaction the child found so useful and enjoyable in the mother.

"The value of touch in human relationships should not be underestimated. From the time the child becomes too proud to be rocked in its mother's arms he does not have the pleasure of close touch again until he arrives at some of the petting of adolescence. Later in marriage each person can be the giver of touch. Neither has to be wholly parent, neither wholly child. But each gives to the other in the play of lovemaking and the sexual relationship."

You need this warmth of touch now more than ever. You need it to keep warm yourself and to generate in you a warmth you can convey to others as you go along.

The Renewal of the Faithful Pact

A fine description of the role of sex at maturity comes from Dr. Martin Gumpert, a Viennese doctor.

Dr. Gumpert said: "There is no greater or more exciting adventure than for two people in love to grow old together. The deepening of wrinkles causes no suffering. Sex becomes a mutual exchange of affection, something both spiritual and animal, and the partner who feels less pleasure will still enjoy the renewal of the faithful pact."

The renewal of the faithful pact! I know of no place where sex at maturity has been more beautifully described.

Many years ago I was coming down in the bus from Stamford, New York, to Poughkeepsie. Opposite me sat a middle-aged couple of sixty or sixty-five. He was tall and soft-boned and stooped, with that peculiar stoop of the European who wasn't trained to exercise in his youth. His face was soft and intelligent too. And his wife was also soft-looking, a small, quiet woman with reddish hair turning gray.

We got to talking. As I had suspected, they were recent refugees. It was the old, old story of the nightmare flight from Hitler, into Switzerland, into France, into Portugal, into a hidden ship by night, and finally to America where they could take a deep breath and start again. It wasn't easy at their age. He had been a distinguished lawyer; now he was glad to find a job as a house-to-house salesman of books. There were times, he told me, when he was in such despair he thought his only job was to deliver his wife here, then lie down and die.

But he hadn't died. Instead, together they were going on.

But what struck me most about them was the way every few minutes he would lean over and gently stroke her hair. It wasn't beautiful hair and she wasn't a beautiful woman, nor had she ever been. But he loved this woman, still loved her tenderly and wholly. I would guess that this quiet couple who had been through so much together still "renewed the faithful pact" of the sex act. It continued to keep them warm and vital, and to give them the courage to go on.

10

You Can Keep Your Figure

Ogden Nash said it:

> *Some ladies smoke too much and*
> *some ladies drink too much*
> *and some ladies pray too much*
> *But all ladies think they weigh too much.*

Menopausal ladies think so especially! We think we weigh too much by far.

In childhood we seldom think about our weight. But in our teens we start to worry. In our twenties and thirties, we worry harder. And by the forties we are wailing long and loud about "that awful middle-aged spread."

Some of us blame the spread on the menopause. "All your glands stop dead during the menopause" is the way one woman explains it. "So of course you *just naturally* get fat as a result." Or we blame it on advancing years in general. "You just have to get fat as you get older" is the way another woman puts it. "And there's nothing you can do about it—nothing at all."

Sorry, ladies, you're wrong. A woman does not just naturally get fat during the menopause. And if she does, there is something she can do about it. Middle-aged spread is not an unkind fate to be accepted like a visitation from the Lord.

Changed Emotions

What is causing the spread? Many things.

Changed emotions for one. Emotional factors are now known to be among the chief villains behind weight gain. Emotional factors such as your new family situation. The loss or threatened loss of your children. A tired marriage or no marriage. Your whole changed pattern of life. You may, for example, be eating more now out of sheer nervousness. Or boredom. Or as a compensation for other things you miss.

Then there may also be plain, everyday factors. The fact that at maturity you *like* to eat more. You have *time* to eat more. You have built up the *habit* of eating more. And perhaps you can *afford* to eat more.

Add all these together—nervousness, compensation, boredom, habit, more money, more time—and you can find yourself nibbling the whole day long. Reaching compulsively for the inner comfort of food much as a drunkard reaches for the inner comfort of drink.

The Inner Comfort of Food

That's a challenging phrase—the "inner comfort of food."

I met a woman not long ago who typified it. She was fortyish, and at one time must have had an excellent figure, for she was tall and carried herself well. But now her suit jacket wouldn't close and her skirt barely spanned her hips.

We happened to be tablemates at a vacation resort for a few weeks and I noticed that at each meal she took seconds on everything. Yet at the same time she kept moaning about how heavy she had grown.

When I asked her how come she was eating so much if her weight worried her, she replied: "I'm overeating because I am worried. My husband died a short time ago and left me quite penniless; I haven't yet decided which way to turn. Meanwhile,

I'm giving myself comfort and filling up the void he left by eating my head off. You might say I'm escaping to the icebox. Well, I suppose I am."

Another heavy woman I knew who worried about her weight still had a husband, but he was out of a job, and she was working as a part-time saleswoman in a department store. She told me that when she was through at four o'clock each day she couldn't resist going into a coffee shop for coffee and a cake, though she'd had a good lunch, and supper was coming along soon. "I know I shouldn't," she confided. "But I work so hard, and I'm so blue in general, that I feel life owes me something, if only a lot of coffee and cake. When my husband gets a job again, I'm sure I'll be able to get off my eating jag."

And a third woman I know put it in a nutshell. "Whenever anything goes wrong, even for a minute, I eat. I eat to comfort myself," she said.

BUT I'M DIFFERENT

"But I'm different," you retort. "I don't eat for comfort. I really need a lot of extra food to help me through my menopause. Besides, I'm sure my body instinctively knows the amount I need."

Well, sorry again, but the argument "I need a lot extra" doesn't hold water either. You may need a *little* extra, but not a lot extra. Yet women use that same excuse in pregnancy, as Addie did: Addie was a businesswoman until she was in her thirties, and until that time was exceedingly careful of her figure. But then along came marriage and pregnancy. She hopped right on the pie-à-la-mode wagon, laughingly passing it off with the old argument that she was "eating for two." Result? Her son is seven years old now, but Addie is still twenty-six pounds overweight.

Alas, nobody knows by instinct the exact amount of food she needs, any more than most animals know. We like to think that animals know, and give as an example the rat, which, throughout its life, eats just about the right amount. But on the other hand there's the guinea pig. A guinea pig in captivity will stuff itself with everything you set before it, stuff itself until it even loses its strong sex drive and doesn't care a hoot whether the whole guinea-pig race lives or dies.

So it looks as though the act of eating is instinctive, but not the amount. When it comes to amount we have to use our heads and deliberately change with the changing years.

Can't we, however, instinctively crave a certain kind of food? Can't we have a natural craving for, say, sugar? Don't we sometimes get such a sugar hunger we just naturally want to eat sweets all day? And doesn't that prove we need sweets at that particular time?

Well, it proves we *want* sweets certainly. But that we need them is something else again. A woman may have a terrific craving for sweets and think she "needs" them, until she finds out she is ill.

There is an illness called hypoglycemia, for instance, that is just the opposite of diabetes. In diabetes the body makes too little insulin. In hypoglycemia it makes too much insulin. As a result a person is always hungry, especially for sugar, since sugar gives the extra insulin something to do.

However, according to Dr. Raphael Kurzrock, if a woman's body makes extra insulin that doesn't mean that she should eat all the sugar she wants. Because if she does, it can become one of those vicious circles: The more sugar she eats, the more insulin her body tends to make, hence the more sugar she wants, and so on. The only answer is for her to eat more meat or other protein. Meat will satisfy her hunger yet not cause all that extra insulin to be made.

So you see you can't always trust a "natural craving for sugar" either.

SWEETS MOSTLY HABIT

There's only one thing to be said about sugar—it tastes good. The passion for sweets is mostly habit—a habit that started when we were very young.

The pleasures of sweets are among our first memories. When we are born we let out a yell and what happens? Somebody quiets us by feeding us sweet milk from a breast or bottle. A little later we start our first adventure with solid food with cereal; and cereal, being starch, turns to sugar in our insides, while for good measure there may be even more sugar on top. (Read the list of ingredients on all the cereal boxes in your supermarket. I did. Out of twenty-four boxes I found only two that didn't list sugar first!) Then, when a birthday rolls around, there is a sweet cake with sweeter icing piled high. While Sunday, Fourth of July, school graduation—any and every important occasion—calls for ice cream and cookies at the very least.

As we grow older this goes on and on. We eat cake at charity bazaars, club meetings, church suppers—eat cake and gossip simultaneously, and come home not remembering which we enjoyed the more. And when even a routine social call becomes boring, what does the hostess do to revive interest? She serves pie or cake.

Is there any wonder, then, that there's an especially strong pull toward sweets during the menopause, when all life can suddenly seem boring or stressful? That we can find ourselves escaping to the candy counter not so much from hunger as from an unconscious desire to sink back into old happy times?

I remember a woman named Sally.

Sally had been a traveling housewares demonstrator for years, and until her forties enjoyed her job thoroughly. But after a while boredom got her, especially evenings in a strange city when she found herself at a loss for what to do. She didn't particularly like the movies, and after a while she seemed to have gotten "all read out," so she slipped into the habit of picking out the best restaurant in town and ordering the richest meal there, mostly to while away the time until she was ready to go to bed. "That big meal killed a full two hours every evening," Sally declared. Result? It also killed her figure. She became almost as broad as she was high.

Make Your Choice

Now I'm not telling you all this as a lecture. If you're much overweight, it's a sore subject, and you've probably lectured yourself blue. Nor am I going to fling at you the grim statistics offered by life insurance companies: how undereaters live through operations easier, get less high blood pressure, and the like.

I'm not going to do any of this because it's your life and your figure, and if you would rather eat everything in sight and stay fair and fat instead of svelte and stylish, then you're surely old enough to know what you want.

But I licked middle-aged spread, and if you want to, you probably can too.

I licked it though I'm less than five feet tall, and five pounds on me shows like fifteen pounds on someone else. I did it though for years I had sworn I "ate like a bird," and my overweight was a mysterious thing I just couldn't understand.

I did it by going to a doctor, taking a deep breath, and plunging. It wasn't easy in spite of all the books that say it is. But the point is—it worked.

My doctor was a Park Avenue, New York, man who specialized in slenderizing actresses and other fashionable women, and I won't mention his name because he charged me a whopping sum for a month's consultation, and all he did for my money was to give me a simple plan, then see me once a week and scream at me if I'd eaten anything I shouldn't. And I mean *scream!* He acted as if I'd committed a murder and literally stormed. But this was mostly an act. Anyway, it was worth it, because he changed my whole way of eating. Better than that, he put into my hands a tool I can use for the rest of my life.

He called this tool a "plan" rather than a "diet list," because diet lists are dreadful things. Diet itself is a horrible word; most of us hate the very sound of it. And as for diet lists, they are often almost impossible to follow. On the day lobster or broccoli is called for, there's neither lobster nor broccoli for miles around. On the day steak or roast beef is called for, steak and roast beef have gone sky high.

But he sat down with me and analyzed my old habits of eating, then gave me new general ideas instead. These general ideas included what I liked to eat and what was available; then he explained how different foods work.

As a starter he made me keep a record for a week of everything I was eating. I had to be honest and write down every single thing. Then we figured out why I'd been eating the things I had and how I could change.

What I wrote down was this:

For breakfast I'd been having fruit and coffee.

For lunch, if I was out, I'd been having only an ice-cream soda. If I was home, some icebox leftovers or a sandwich with mayonnaise, and tea with lemon and sugar.

In the middle of the afternoon I'd sneaked in tea and crackers or cake.

For supper, meat, vegetables, and dessert.

"Why," I asked him with the usual skepticism, "had I been getting fat on *that?*"

Analyzing My Breakfast

He said he'd take up everything in due course. First, my breakfast.

My breakfast, he pointed out, was an entirely wrong way to start a day. Even though I wanted to lose weight, I needed more for breakfast. I needed to add to my fruit and coffee a little bulk in the form of a dish of cereal, an egg, or a slice of toast, preferably whole grain, with cottage cheese instead of butter on it. This bulk was to keep me going through the morning, and prevent me from getting so hungry that I grabbed the first thing that popped in front of my eyes—the soda if I was out, the leftovers if I was home.

He also pointed out something quite surprising about having a slice of toast for breakfast. This was that I must on no account add jelly to the toast. "Why?" I interrupted. "If I'm supposed to have a little more breakfast to keep me going, isn't jelly just the energy food I need?" "No," he answered firmly. "The trouble with jelly is, it gives too much energy. Does its job too well. Jelly for breakfast can give you such a big spurt of energy that your blood sugar soars way up around eleven o'clock. Then, as a reaction, about eleven-thirty your blood sugar falls way down low.

This can leave you ravenous for lunch at noon. But if you have coffee and an egg for breakfast, or coffee and plain cereal or toast, your blood sugar stays more constant. Your morning energy may thus last longer, and you may not need nearly so much lunch."

Analyzing My Lunch

Now as to the lunch itself. Why had I been snatching at that silly ice-cream soda? Or those almost as silly icebox leftovers? What was behind this?

Well, I answered, now that I thought it over, it was mistaken busyness, or laziness. I was snatching at a soda when I was in town because I was too busy, or thought I was, to sit down in a restaurant. And at home I was too lazy to have the proper food in the house or to prepare a decent lunch. Slapping some filling between two chunks of bread, or grabbing some cold spaghetti, was by far the easiest way out.

At this point he surprised me again by saying that if I weren't so lazy or busy I could eat almost twice as much lunch as I had been yet still lose weight. But first I'd have to have a lesson on calories. Calories are humdrum scientific things that measure how different foods act. But humdrum or not, they make you thin or fat.

A person my height needs at most fifteen hundred calories a day to maintain weight, he said, and has to dip down to a thousand calories or less to lose. (Some people can lose on fifteen hundred a day, but not me.) Did I realize that an ice-cream soda accounted for three hundred and fifty of the calorie allotment right off the reel? And a sandwich, what with butter or mayonnaise on it, did the same? Yes, ma'am, three hundred fifty calories right there for either soda or sandwich—a full third of the day's ration though I still thought I was "eating like a bird."

Sad but true, he told me, if I wanted to reduce I'd have to start to count my calories. If I didn't count, my stomach would!

Luckily, however, after I digested two basic ideas this counting wasn't particularly hard to do.

The two basic ideas were these: There are friendly foods and enemy foods.

Fats and starches are the arch enemies of keep-your-figure people, fats even more than starches. They're enemies because they contain the most calories for the amount of "staying power" they have. That is, fats and starches give a lot of immediate satisfaction, but, as we saw in the case of the jelly, they don't stay with you long.

On the other hand, proteins, fruits, and vegetables are the friends of keep-your-figure people. Proteins because they contain the least amount of calories for their staying power; fruits and vegetables because they contain few calories altogether as a rule.

THE FRIENDLY FOODS

The friendly proteins are things such as lean meats, fish, eggs, and plain cheeses such as cottage cheese. It always shocks people to learn that some cheeses are on the mustn't touch list. But it stands to reason that if cream cheese, for instance, contains cream, it's fattening, isn't it? And cheeses such as roquefort and cheddar have high fat contents too.

The friendly vegetables are the green vegetables such as string beans and cabbage, and yellow vegetables such as carrots and squash. Potatoes, if you leave the butter off them, aren't half so bad as most folks think. Actually, baked beans and corn, which always come dressed up with butter or fat, are much worse than the potato whose reputation is so bad.

The friendly fruits are fruits such as oranges, apples, and berries eaten plain. The exceptions among fruits are bananas which are bursting with starch (although they are good sources of potassium); and dried fruits bursting with sugar such as apricots, prunes, or grapes from which raisins are made.

THE ENEMY FOODS

The enemy fats for figure keepers are bacon, butter, cream, nuts, and fat meats such as pork. Nuts are another shocker. Men especially think nuts are innocent, and they can nibble at them the evening long. But being full of fat, nuts are positively dynamite, which of course includes peanut butter, too, as well as another surprise—the skin of poultry. Give the skin to your dog, who'll be very grateful.

The enemy starches are things such as spaghetti, rice, noodles, pancakes, and bread. Certainly there is a "starch-reduced" spaghetti. But there is no such thing as a "nonfattening" spaghetti. Starch-reduced means there is maybe twenty percent less starch, which leaves eighty percent starch if my arithmetic is right. And eighty percent is a great big lot. Though to a certain extent bread and crackers, as we'll see in a moment, are a far worse enemy than spaghetti. Spaghetti tempts most of us only occasionally. Bread and crackers are always around. What's more, bread and crackers never seem to count.

And of course desserts such as pies, cakes, and puddings, since they contain both fats and starches, are in the enemy class— though I actually met a man who thought rice pudding wasn't fattening! It just goes to show you never can tell what people will believe.

A Quick Calorie Counter

Now as to the actual calories.

My doctor pointed out that I didn't have to know the calorie value of every food; nobody ever did. But if I remembered the important ones, these would do. Here are the main ones to keep in mind:

An average piece of bread, no matter whether
white or dark, plain or toast (in toast, all that's
been dried out is the water) equals . . . .   75 calories
A small pat of butter . . . .   <u>25</u>   "
So an average slice of bread and butter
equals   100   "

An average cracker equals 25   "

$$\times 4$$

So four crackers are about the same as a piece
of bread and butter 100   "

BUT an average serving of meat, with much
more staying power than a slice of bread and
butter or four crackers, is only . . . . . 150 calories
Two average eggs (staying power again) . . 150   "
An average glass of milk 75   "
An average serving of green vegetables . . 50   "
One shrimp, oyster, or scallop (hurrah)
only 10   "
One small piece of pie, or layer cake, or
double-scoop ice-cream soda, that awful . . 350   "

So, starting to count calories, and getting back to my lunch,
here's what I could do: I could have two satisfying eggs (one
hundred and fifty calories) plus a large serving of a green vegetable such as string beans (fifty calories), and total only two hundred calories, or about half as much as the ice-cream soda I often
took. What's more, on the same principle as no jelly for breakfast, no sugar for lunch would keep me going far better during
the afternoon.

Or instead of the eggs I could have a hearty oyster stew for
lunch and still total only two hundred calories again (one hundred calories for the ten oysters, plus seventy-five for the hot
milk, plus another twenty-five for the pat of butter dropped in).
Yet an oyster stew would also "stay with" me all afternoon, so I
probably would not even desire afternoon crackers with tea.

And of course I could have a broiled hamburger without the
bun (whose purpose is mainly to make it look thicker), or cottage cheese and a salad for lunch. In fact, cottage cheese, like the
much-talked-about yogurt, is a mainstay of figure keepers. They
get to rely on it like their good right hand.

All this, my doctor repeated, depended on my getting over
my laziness about lunch. I'd have to plan to buy the right foods
in advance and have them on hand. But luckily eggs and cottage

cheese, and hamburger are everywhere available. And oysters and shrimp (those blessed ten-calorie objects) are now almost everywhere available also.

Analyzing My Dinner

Dinner is usually easier to plan than lunch. As to dinner, therefore, I'd been doing pretty well. The fish I'd been eating was fine, as long as I broiled it or baked it. The meat was also fine, as long as I remembered to cut the fat off before I brought it to the table.

Never forget that fat is the most fattening food there is. One gram of protein or starch equals four calories; one gram of fat nine calories. So, beware: Substitute for dessert, fruit with a teaspoon of half-and-half cream on it if it is fresh fruit, or a teaspoon of sugar on it if it has been cooked.

At this point, having analyzed what I'd been doing wrong, my doctor proceeded to make his careful-eating plan still simpler. He boiled it down to a Rule of Three, a rule which called for hardly any strain on my memory, and which I could apply anywhere and any time.

Here is his Rule of Three:

At each meal I could eat three main things:

- a *protein,* such as meat, fish, or eggs;
- a *starch,* such as one slice of bread, or four crackers, or one plain potato;
- a *green vegetable,* or a piece of *frest fruit;*

and coffee or tea with a little whole milk in them. (There's so little fat in the amount of milk you put in coffee or tea, it really doesn't count.)

You apply the rule like this, or make up your own similar combinations:

BREAKFAST BY THE RULE OF THREE

Orange juice	(fruit)
Scrambled egg	(protein)
Small plate of cereal	(starch)

Coffee with milk   (doesn't count)
  or
Grapefruit   (fruit)
Grilled lean ham   (protein)
Slice of toast   (starch)
Coffee with milk   (doesn't count)

LUNCH BY THE RULE OF THREE

Oyster stew   (protein)
Mixed green salad   (vegetable)
Crackers   (starch)
  or
Tuna fish   (protein)
Melba toast   (starch)
Baked apple, homemade   (fruit)
  with minimum of sugar
  or
Hamburger   (protein)
Half a bun   (starch)
Stewed plums   (fruit)
Tea with lemon   (doesn't count)

DINNER BY THE RULE OF THREE

Lamb chops   (protein)
Parsleyed boiled potato   (starch)
Cauliflower   (vegetable)
Coffee with milk   (doesn't count)
  or
Broiled calves' liver   (protein)
Baked potato   (starch)
Honeydew melon   (fruit)
Coffee with milk   (doesn't count)
  or
Halibut steak   (protein)
Slice of bread   (starch)

| Parsleyed carrots | (vegetable) |
| Tea with milk | (doesn't count) |

Everything for Health

Having given me this Rule of Three, my doctor proceeded to point out something else that was good to hear. Not only was his plan simple and easy to follow, it included everything I needed to keep me in excellent general health. It contained abundant protein, which is the prime body-builder and restorer; vegetables and fruits for natural vitamins; coffee and tea as the mild stimulants which older people need; and whole milk for nourishment to teeth, skin, and bones. If in addition I added to it a daily all-purpose vitamin, preferably one with calcium in it, then I would be well taken care of.

On the other hand, to get back to those ever-tempting sweets such as pie and cake, they were really "kid stuff." No adult needs them. However, if I simply had to have some for inner comfort and inner comfort can be important too—then he suggested I make a small piece of pie or cake a once-a-week treat. But only once a week, mind you, or I'd undo all my other good work. Once a week, therefore, if I kept to his plan the rest of the time, I could give myself a reward—a reward to keep up my morale and make me feel I was still like folks. A reward to prevent me from talking about myself. If there's one person other people don't like to have around, it's someone who eats differently than they do and keeps talking about it. So to keep my popularity, maybe the best idea was to save my weekly treat for the evening I was invited out. Then I could join the others around the table without calling attention to myself, for which everybody would give thanks.

Calories as an Allowance

Having imbibed this much wisdom, I took another deep breath and plunged. I tried to do as the doctor told me—consider my calories as an allowance, like youngsters consider their pocket money. That is, if I spent my money on extra potatoes one day, I'd have no money left for bread, and so on down the line. It was worth it, though, because it worked. I hurried back to his office a week after my first visit, stepped on the scales, and found I'd lost a pound. He'd told me that for a person my size and weight a pound a week was all I could expect. A pound doesn't sound like much, but it went in proportion. If I'd been taller, or started out, say, twenty pounds overweight, I might have expected to lose two pounds a week. But five pounds a week as some diet schemes promise? It can't be done. Or if it can be done, it shouldn't be. Two pounds a week should be tops for any woman, and a pound was tops for me.

But the next week, on the same number of calories, I didn't even lose that pound. I lost only half a pound. And the week following I lost nothing at all! I almost cried until he told me this might also be expected.

Indeed, I almost changed my resolution to "eat, drink, and be merry, for tomorrow we diet." Always that eternal tomorrow. But I changed back again when he explained that, for some curious reason, no matter what one does, weight loss is not constant. It comes in fits and spurts.

To cheer me up, he told me about a series of experiments done at the University of Michigan. A Mrs. Andrews was put on fifteen hundred calories a day instead of her usual twenty-three hundred. This meant eight hundred calories less, or a reduction of a third of her usual amount. Yet did she lose regularly? She didn't. In spite of the fact that she was kept under strict supervision and couldn't possibly cheat, she lost weight for the first two days, stayed exactly the same for the next ten days, then began to lose again, and finally ended down.

Then a Mrs. Whitney on a similar regimen didn't lose at all for the first sixteen days. While a Mr. Hart actually weighed more after his first five days of dieting than before. Though at last he began to lose, gained again, lost again, and finally ended down.

My doctor's moral was to be persistent. Also, not to look ahead; to think only of today. For if a woman decides to lose as much as forty pounds, and looks ahead to the months it may take her to do it, she'll be discouraged before she starts. But lose one to two pounds a week, even in fits and starts, and think *only* of those one to two pounds? O.K.

The successful members of Alcoholics Anonymous, he said, have learned this same lesson. They never promise themselves, "I won't take a drink for a year," since a year sounds endless, and it's a promise they maybe could not keep. Instead, they say each morning: "I won't take a drink *today.*"

Some Fine Points

"And if you really want to get down and stay down, there are some even finer points you might want to know," the doctor went on.

One was about chocolate; another about alcohol; another about oranges versus grapefruit; and still another about salt.

- *Chocolate twice as villainous as vanilla*
  About chocolate: Chocolate is more than twice as bad as vanilla as a weight producer. A scoop of chocolate ice cream adds up to two and one half times as many calories as a ball of vanilla ice cream, for the simple reason that chocolate contains a lot of fat.

- *Sweet wines more fattening than dry wines*
  About alcohol: All alcohol is fattening, because alcohol is full of calories; and alcohol causes a craving for more food. But hard liquor, such as in a mixed drink, is far more fattening than light wine; and as far as wine is concerned, dry wine, such as Rhine wine or chablis, is much better than sweet wine such as sherry or port, because sweet wine contains more sugar.

  So you may enjoy a little light wine with your dinner, if you remember to count the calories in it when you plan your food allowance, since light wine, especially as you grow older, can be relaxing. But stay away from cocktails and beer as you would from the plague. Women often laugh at a man's "beer belly." Well, women can develop a "beer belly" or a "cocktail belly," too.

- *Oranges twice as fattening as grapefruit*

About oranges: They are twice as fattening as grapefruit, because of the natural sugar in oranges. A glass of orange juice jumps up to a hundred calories, but a glass of grapefruit juice only half as much.

- *Salt can be a hidden enemy*

And salt is almost as fattening as sugar.

This was surprising to me when the doctor pronounced it, and may be equally surprising to you. But many older women, it seems, are waterlogged. Much of their excess weight is plain water. And salt helps the body to retain water. If they get rid of the water, ergo, they get rid of the weight. If they keep the water with the aid of salt, they keep the weight.

That didn't mean, of course, I couldn't use a small amount of salt in cooking to make my food palatable. But it did mean leaving out every speck of extra salt at the table. Also things such as anchovies, pickles, ketchup, chili sauce, and condiments of every kind.

Yes, he knew, I might be devoted to pickles and condiments. Leaving them out might be harder than anything else. But there it was: the salt in them could keep me good and fat. Also, condiments are very irritating to the intestines, and the intestines in older people are more sensitive than in younger ones.

So I took another deep breath and reluctantly changed my occasional treat from chocolate ice cream to vanilla (or strawberry, or pineapple, but not walnut. I switched from sherry to sauterne, orange juice to grapefruit, and cut down as much as possible on salt.

It took just about a month and I'd done it—lost those horrible pounds that had rested on my middle for years. People began to pay me so many compliments, I thought of my dentist, who insists the nicest words in the English language are, "Enclosed find check!" Oh no, they aren't, I said to myself. They are, "You did it. You said you would, and you did."

But now thinner, I had one of those hindsight brain waves. Why all the bother in the first place? Couldn't I have merely bought myself some reducing drugs instead?

Reducing drugs, I argued with my doctor, have a most appealing sound. Why can't you just eat all you want, then take a pill?

Well, he answered, let's look at what's available. Thyroid pills? Yes. Thyroid pills do help some people. But they help only after careful tests have shown they need them. If you take them when you don't need them, they may do you no good. Worse, even small doses of thyroid taken when you don't need them may slow up your own thyroid to where you'll find yourself back where you started. Large doses tend to pile up in your system, and weeks or months later you may get the jitters and wonder why. "Do you want to risk the jitters?" he asked me. "No," I answered, "I definitely do not."

Next, there's benzedrine. Or its cousin dexadrine. A "benny" taken about an hour before mealtime certainly may give you a lift and take away some of the desire for food. But benzedrine and dexadrine can be even more potent drugs than thyroid; they can really give you the jitters. Also, they only work for a few weeks, then stop. On top of this, they are highly addictive. Did I want to risk addiction? I answered again with a firm "no."

Or as another doctor, Dr. Charles Birnberg of the Brooklyn Jewish Hospital, once laughingly put it to me: "If there were any decent reducing drugs, wouldn't I know about them? And if I did, would I be as fat as I am?"

A Matter of Habit

So keeping your figure at the menopause comes back to where we started—mainly eating the right food, and learning to enjoy the right food when you eat it.

Enjoying the right food is important because if you want to keep down after you've gotten down, you'll have to be careful of what you eat for the rest of your life. That's why nine-day diets are no good, or eighteen-day diets, or any other kind of trick stunt. They're useless unless you keep up the good work.

And keeping it up means forming new habits. Learning to *like* meat and vegetables instead of starches. To run past the candy store with the scrumptious display in the window. To fly past the bakery with the alluring smells. To ask yourself frankly: Am I nibbling mostly from boredom or whatever? And if so get away from the source of temptation—fast.

Studies have shown that women with outside jobs are thinner than those who stay home. Why? The home-stayers constantly have food around to tempt them; the outside-jobbers do not. The moral again: when tempted to "nosh" or snack between meals, get out for a walk or an errand where you'll meet neighbors. Or call a friend on the phone and keep talking until the temptation goes.

HOW TO ENJOY VEGETABLES

As a tip for enjoying vegetables, the best thing that ever crossed my path is the pressure cooker. After using it for a while I'm sure that many of us don't like vegetables because all our lives we've eaten them so horribly overdone they've become a soggy mess on the plate. But pressured on a rack that keeps them out of water, they're bright and firm and have flavors you never dreamed of. On my recommendation invest in a cooker (it's cheaper than outsize clothes), and try cabbage, broccoli, carrots, or brussels sprouts. They're so good that my husband, who loathed vegetables as only a man can, began to beg for two portions.

And please believe me when I say that pressure cookers don't explode when you handle them properly. In fact, I'm so sold on them for delicious vegetables and stews and potroasts, even fish steaks, that I own two of them—a big one and a little one. Or if you don't like pressure cookers, try a vegetable-steamer, which also keeps the vegetables out of water and saves the vitamins. You'll have no need for vitamin pills.

HOW TO ENJOY COFFEE WITH MILK

As another tip for enjoying coffee with milk instead of cream, try *café au lait* made the French way. That is, very fresh, very strong coffee mixed half and half with hot milk. Heating milk almost but not quite to the boiling point seems to thicken it and "do something" to it. The French then pour coffee and milk simultaneously into the cup, so that they mix as they pour. Delicious! Try it once or twice; you'll probably never go back to coffee with cream.

However, stick to whole milk, not skim milk. Dr. Celia Bercow tells me of the fashionable women who come to her office with their skins all dry and taut from substituting skim milk for whole milk. Whole milk contains fat in the form of natural vitamin A, which you need to nourish and beautify your skin. So don't leave it completely out, especially as you get older.

THE NUMBERS GAME

Still, whole milk or skim, as you grow older you will have to learn to play the food-numbers game.

Here's why:

Metabolism, as you know, is the process by which we burn food, and calories are the units of measurement that express the amount of heat burned by food as it passes through the body. But metabolism and calorie-burning change with the years. During the first year of life when we are practically doubling in size and weight, we eat and burn calories like mad. But as growth slows down, eating and burning slow down: a child proportionately eats less than a baby. But then around age ten both our appetites and our rate of calorie burning perk up, and around age fifteen they perk up again as we reach for our full height. But after fifteen there's another change. Now there is a steady and permanent slowing down.

George Washington University's Dr. Herbert Pollack, former chairman of the Nutrition Committee of the American Heart Association, says this is how the slowing down works out:

At the age of fifteen, an active girl five feet two inches tall weighing one hundred twenty-five pounds can burn sixteen hundred calories a day. In her twenties she can burn only thirteen hundred seventy calories a day. In her thirties thirteen hundred calories, and by her forties and fifties, much, much less.

This lessened use is due in part, to a slowing down in activity. At fifteen, a girl is playing hard, swimming, dancing, batting a tennis ball, taking long hikes. By the time she is twenty-five, she has slowed down to being an office worker, a housekeeper, or some other mainly sit-down job. By thirty-five, she may be a busier housekeeper and worker, but she no longer wants to wash, sweep, and scrub by hand. If she can possibly manage it, she's the possessor of an automatic washing machine, a vacuum cleaner, an electric cake mixer, and an electric dishwasher. By forty-five she has probably acquired a car with automatic shift and power steering, and she seldom walks to any place to which she can ride. A Stamford, New York, woman told me it was good that she had indoor plumbing instead of a privy, because otherwise she might find herself backing up her car to get to it.

Is it any wonder, then, that if we continue to eat as much at thirty-five or forty-five as we did at fifteen, our pounds mount up and our figure spreads?

COMPLEX REASONS

Women who do continue to eat as much usually do so for complex reasons. This is because eating is far from simple.

At first a baby eats mainly to survive. But soon taking in food also becomes a way of getting loved—cuddled at the breast if breast-fed, held in its mother's arms if bottle-fed.

As she grows, the desire for love becomes stronger. But now it is love for herself. As soon as she can, a small girl does what her mother originally did for her—gets love through food. She buys herself an ice-cream cone. She goes to parties not only for sociability but because a main attraction is the fact that she can devour a special party cake down to the last delicious crumb.

During adolescence eating has become still more complicated. Now there have been added the elements of belonging, anxiety, and revolt. Many of the rich foods on which a teenager gorges make her so full she forgets to be afraid. She eats others because they make her feel part of the crowd, or were formerly forbidden. The zesty pizza pies savored in the dorm at midnight, the bacon and onion sandwiches munched before a bonfire, the double-fudge sundaes held for extra minutes on the tongue: these are doubly alluring because for the first time in her life she can rebel and eat as she pleases or as the crowd pleases, and she indulges to the hilt. So adolescence is a peak of eating pleasure, with survival, belonging, anxiety, and revolt all mixed in together, as a teenager lives almost literally from hand to mouth.

By the time a woman is grown, these factors have so added up that eating has become incredibly complex, especially when old feelings connected with food well up. Then an adult may find herself turning to ways of satisfying them that have nothing to do with real needs.

There was Eleanor, for instance, who always felt her younger and cuter sister got all the attention in the family. In her teens, whenever her sister had a date and she didn't, Eleanor was so miserable she ate and ate, until she ran straight up to one hundred seventy-five pounds. She stayed there until she realized that she ate mainly from jealousy, got the courage to reduce, and because she was thinner began to date herself. And when she got married, did she have a splashy wedding! Though after that, since she had now become a compulsive eater, she again went up and down.

Many older people keep up this habit of eating, for emotional reasons. So do some musicians and actors after a performance, both to unwind and, particularly if they're not certain they've done well, to reassure themselves. When Maria Callas was a young and struggling singer, she used to eat a whole pound of cheese at a sitting. When she became successful, she was more or less able to stop. She, too, though, was a compulsive eater and one time when she was heavy, she did a strange thing: A man who dressed her hair at the Metropolitan Opera told me how she had a doctor give her a tapeworm to swallow, then later had him give her medicine to get rid of the tapeworm, but only after she had lost eighty pounds.

MORE EMOTIONAL FACTORS

Great weight-gain in us more ordinary people is also common after the emotional jolt of the death of a beloved relative or friend. And the poor notoriously eat more than the rich. The poor eat because expensive forms of entertainment are not readily available to them, so every holiday calls for a feast. And many people eat to "keep up their strength," forgetting that unnecessary food actually taxes their strength by all the extra work it gives their bodies to do to digest it.

As to eating for revolt, this can continue, too. One of the surest ways to get a woman to eat for revolt is to have a doctor or member of her family force a diet on her. Then, like the drunkard who hides his whiskey in the bathroom cabinet because his wife wants him to sober up, she'll hide chocolate bars under her pillow, or clean up everything in the refrigerator, from sheer spite. This determination to eat what one wants to is the basis, also, for much of the griping about hospital food. Hospital authorities usually buy the best foodstuff obtainable, but the patient feels she is a prisoner and didn't choose it, so she refuses to enjoy the food no matter how much the staff tries.

DESIRE FOR LOVE

Probably the biggest factor in overeating is the desire to buy oneself love. Women who feel unloved often do their extra eating in restaurants, where waiters, whom they tip generously, hover about them and the proprietor beams as he anticipates the huge check. A fifty-two-year-old woman who habitually ate in restaurants said that at such times she fancied herself a queen surrounded by her grateful court.

Then there was the famous and beautiful actress Maxine Elliott. Speaking about Maxine in her autobiography, Elsa Maxwell says, "It didn't seem fair for so much brains and beauty to be wrapped up in one woman." But Elsa went on to tell how Maxine disappeared from the stage at the height of her fame and Elsa found her in her Riviera villa sitting by the side of her pool, enormously fat and eating nonstop. It seems that Maxine had fallen in love with a young Australian tennis player many years her junior, and when he suddenly died, making her lose his love, she started to eat as compulsively as a chain-smoker smokes.

Though her doctor warned her it would kill her—and it did—she couldn't stop.

The singer Judy Garland went on eating binges when she was unhappy, too, ordering huge hotel meals sent up to her room at 3 A.M. The studio had forbidden her to eat very much when she was a child star; now she swung from diets to eating binges, and her weight went up and down so violently she seemed like a lost little girl in an adult world.

Then there's the compulsion many women have to eat up the leftovers while doing the dishes. They will take an extra roll, a scrap of meat, an end of piecrust neither they nor anyone else wanted at the table, and hastily swallow it with the excuse, "I can't bear to throw anything out." Instead, they throw it in. They keep on doing this for years, then wail in astonishment, "How can I have gotten so fat when I eat like a bird?"

MORE ARITHMETIC

Here's one way they've done it:

Says Dr. Rachmeil Levine: for every pound of weight you gain, you gain another three-quarters of a pound of water which the fat cells hold in your body. Keep on doing this indefinitely; the thought is staggering!

Luckily, however, there's something that steps in and partly stops this process. This is the fact that metabolism is dependent, among other things, on the square feet of body surface. If you have a big or tall body you can burn up more than if you have a small body, regardless of your age or work. A big body is in some ways like a robber baron; it demands a lot of tribute. It therefore takes extra calories just to carry a big body around. So if one is really very fat or very tall, one can eat more than a small person can, and not gain as fast. It also works the other way around. When a large woman goes on a diet, she usually complains at first that she is constantly hungry. But once she becomes smaller, her body is not so demanding; it becomes satisfied with less.

A few more happy facts:

Three approximately equal meals a day are less fattening than two small meals and one large—say just coffee for breakfast, a sandwich for lunch and a traditional "good dinner." Experiments have been done with rats divided into two groups called The Nibblers and The Gobblers. The Nibblers got three meals of nearly equal size. The Gobblers got tiny breakfasts and tiny lunches, leaving them so hungry they gobbled up their big dinners. Each group got exactly the same calories; the only difference was the way in which they were divided. The Gobblers gained more. Similar experiments were done with women, with the same results. Gobbling women gained more, too.

There's more to gobbling than eating big dinners, though. There's the matter of how fast food is eaten. Many women afraid of gaining weight get into the habit of bolting whatever they eat, because they are guilty about eating it in the first place, and swallowing it down fast somehow seems to get it out of sight. Unfortunately, this only makes the situation worse. Now they feel guilty about their bad shape.

Dr. William Kroger gives this advice to women who want to keep their figures: "Cut down on all food as you get older. But don't cut out your favorite foods altogether because living should be enjoyable, and eating is an important part of it. In the main, however, eat slowly of delicate things divided into nearly equal meals."

SUGAR NOT "QUICK ENERGY"

It's important, too, to get over the notion that one needs sugar for quick energy. Certainly sugar releases energy quickly, but then so does all food. Sugar releases it maybe fifteen seconds faster, and the only person in whom these fifteen seconds might be crucial is a soldier ready to faint on a forced march, or a diabetic ready to go into a coma from too much insulin. But few of us are soldiers or diabetics. We are ordinary people, and for us a cracker or a piece of cheese will supply whatever quick energy we need.

The craving for sugar, to repeat, is mainly due to the fact that one associates sweets with pleasant memories from the time when they were youthful treats. But a person who got hot dogs or dill pickles as youthful treats can crave dill pickles or hot dogs, and it doesn't prove she "needs" them, either. Besides, there were thousands of years when refined sugar as we know it today was unknown, and people enjoyed the natural fruit-sugars and honey instead. Yet they survived and stayed energetic. They also only got these natural sugars rarely, at certain seasons of the year. Can you imagine the biblical Sarah "needing" fudge-bars so she could go about her labors, when the only memories she had were of fruits or honey a few times a year?

But all life is a going forward and a pulling back. So some women who remember the pleasures of sugar may still want occasionally to slip back into the happy delirium of childhood with such things as a mile-high lemon pie or a shimmering coconut layer-cake. But they should understand these sweets for what they are—special treats for special celebrations, not super-quick energy foods.

Luckily, some women find they actually lose their taste for sweets as they get older. As their metabolism slows down and their chemistry changes, their sugar-craving, if it ever existed, naturally fades away. These women are fortunate because a calorie-allowance is like money in your pocket; you can spend only so much. With sweets eliminated, one can buy more of the meats, fishes, salads, and plain cheeses that are true body-restorers. They can also buy a little more butter, because of the pleasant fact that women's hormones seem to protect their arteries from clogging with cholesterol from fats like butter the way men's get clogged.

Some Weight Tables

Here are some up-to-date tables on desirable weights according to height, compiled by the Metropolitan Life Insurance Company. As you study them, notice as always that normal has wide variations, and that different weights are given for different size frames, since a woman with big bones and wide hips has more places to tuck pounds in than a woman with tiny bones. Notice, too, that age does not count after twenty-five, since an adolescent often tends to be too fat or too thin, but a woman should settle down by twenty-five and then stay about the same until old age. (These are heights and weights taken without shoes.)

Desirable Weights After Age 25

	Small Frame	Medium Frame	Large Frame
4′ 10″	92-98	96-107	104-119
11″	94-101	98-110	106-122
5′ 0″	96-104	101-113	109-125
1″	99-107	104-116	112-128
2″	102-110	107-119	115-131
3″	105-113	110-122	118-134
4″	108-116	113-126	121-138
5″	111-119	116-130	125-142
6″	114-123	120-135	129-146
7″	118-127	124-139	133-150
8″	122-131	128-143	137-154
9″	126-135	132-147	141-158
10″	130-140	136-151	145-163
11″	134-144	140-155	149-168
6′ 0″	138-148	144-159	153-173

Desirable weights, of course, don't take into account fat distribution, the baffling problem of why some women seem to have all their bulges on their thighs and others around their waists. The only answer to this is, they just do. Usually their mothers and grandmothers did before them; the fat in their families simply tends to accumulate there. Experiments have been done in which a chunk of tissue from a woman's fat thighs was transposed onto the back of one of her hands. The back of that hand soon accumulated fat, while the other hand did not. That's why "spot reducing" does no good unless one reduces all over; the bulges tend to come back in the same place. It may make you mad, but there it is.

WHEN NOT TO REDUCE

With all this talk of reducing, there are times not to even try.

One time not to try, says Dr. Hilde Bruch, is during a time of extreme emotional tension, such as when a member of the family is very ill. You can't go by the weight tables at such a time, and if a woman diets to the point where she finds she's always cranky or can't work, she is doing neither herself nor anyone else any good.

"We hear much about the self-indulgence and lack of will power of people who overeat," says Dr. Bruch. "It is rarely recognized that dieting may also be a kind of self-indulgence, a selfish preoccupation with appearance that may breed characteristics that make the dieter unbearable to those around her." Dieting to this point is another form of neurosis—an "all or nothing" attitude that makes the person end up with the loss of love she doesn't want.

That's also the trouble with crash diets. They are so meager they amount to "nothing," so almost no one ever sticks to them unless she lets a doctor lock her up in a hospital. Surveys have shown that sixty-five percent of women who go on crash diets promptly get off them, and at the end of a short time are back where they were before. They have merely wasted their enthusiasm, if they haven't done themselves serious harm.

DIET SPECIALISTS

Since the problems of food and eating are so complex, in the past few years there has been a great increase in the number of diet specialists, as well as diet clinics such as the University of Pennsylvania's Behavioral Weight-Control Clinic. These take a psychological approach to overeating and insist that an analysis of a woman's eating habits, followed by a change in her behavior, is the only way for her to get down and stay down.

The first thing the behavior-specialists do is to ask the people who come to them to keep a food diary. Write down immediately every scrap of food eaten, including such small items as three peanuts or four potato chips, and do it the minute they are eaten. In this way, if they think they are only eating twelve hundred calories a day, they can prove it. If they are eating more, it stares them in the face.

Keeping an immediate diary also slows people down, and makes eating a conscious choice instead of a compulsion. And if they also write down *why* they eat what they do, it reveals the emotional reason behind an eating binge, and lets them work to correct that.

The specialists also point out the value of dieting as a member of a group. "The group is not there to embarrass those who gain, or reward those who lose," says Dr. Leonard Levitz, head of one of the behavioral clinics. "It is there to exchange ideas. People get fat in a million different ways and they lose in a million different ways. And we all need a lot of ideas."

One of the best known groups is *Weight Watchers*. At the first meeting, it asks a woman to set herself a goal, usually a loss of no more than twenty pounds, since a bigger loss sounds frightening. They also tell her that it should take her about three months to lose this much. Three months may sound slow, but it averages out to two pounds a week and they believe that is a maximum. After all, she gained her weight slowly; she should lose it slowly, too. (I gained four pounds on a month-long binge from cookies bought at Christmas bake sales. It took me another month to get them off.)

And of course, say Weight Watchers, get weighed only once a week and at the same time of the day, preferably halfway between two meals. Also use a balance scale. The usual scale is too erratic, especially if kept in the bathroom, where the steam will throw it off. I keep my money in a certain bank just because they have a fine big balance scale.

A FEW TIPS

A recent article in *Cue* magazine offers more practical tips. Here they are:

Don't eat standing up.

When eating at home, eat in the same place, sit down at a table, use small plates and small glasses so the meal won't look so skimpy, because we eat with our eyes as well as our mouths.

When you eat, attend only to eating: don't talk on the phone, watch TV, or cook. Eating while cooking tempts you to "nosh."

Keep a boring refrigerator while dieting. You can pep it up later.

Consume foods you can't resist only at a restaurant, because portions there are controlled. And obviously order à la carte instead of "getting your money's worth" table d'hôte.

Eat food slowly, chew it thoroughly, learn to appreciate its sensory aspects by rolling it on your tongue.

Put utensils down between bites so you won't stuff yourself nonstop.

Never clean your plate on general principles.

Always eat off a plate, even if it's just a single potato chip or carrot stick. That's another way of saying, don't eat standing up.

Shop only from a prepared list. Impulse shopping can be ruinous.

Assume that sometimes you will cheat, some days you will fail. So don't get angry at yourself. Start again.

MORE TIPS

Drink a large glass of a low-calorie carbonated drink fifteen minutes before mealtime. This will take the edge off a too hearty appetite.

If in doubt whether a food contains a lot of fat, use the napkin test. Take a piece of cheese and set it on a paper napkin. If it leaves a greasy spot on the napkin, it is a "no-no."

Don't diet strenuously when you are ill, such as in the midst of a bad headache; it will only make the headache worse. I eat a light meal of hot cereal with a little half-and-half cream over it when I have a headache, and follow that with applesauce, because I know that when my head is aching my stomach is tense also. A meal like this slips down quite easily.

Exercise

So far I haven't said a word about exercise, but the plain truth is if you want to keep your figure, you not only have to stick to a careful diet indefinitely, you also have to exercise. And you can learn to enjoy exercise just as you can learn to enjoy the right food.

The chief trick to learning to enjoy exercise is to do it in a group. Make exercise as much a social thing as a movement thing. Sign up for an exercise class where you'll meet friendly people. Or buy a bike, find a friend with a bike, and go on rides with her. Alone, you'll probably never stick to an exercise schedule, just as practically no one ever sticks to using one of those gimmicky exercycle machines for the simple reason that gimmicks quickly become dull and exercise should be fun.

As to the value of exercise, it will stimulate every cell in your body; it will make your heart work more efficiently; it will increase the capacity of your lungs; it will improve the circulation of blood to your brain. (Yes, it will actually keep your mind from deteriorating.)

Exercise will improve your posture, and as a result will relieve some of the backaches that women in particular suffer from. Then your bones will become stronger and denser and your high blood pressure, if you have any, will be reduced. In other words, exercise will make you feel infinitely better in every way.

Recently the National Administration on Aging did a special study on older people. They took a group of moderately healthy seventy-year-olds who had been doing little more than knit, or sit in a rocking chair while they read their daily papers, and for a year put them through a course of fairly vigorous exercise. At the end of that year the seventy-year-olds had the general body-reactions of thirty-year-olds. To be sure, they didn't exactly look like thirty-year-olds, but no one had expected they would. But they did feel more like thirty-year-olds. And what could be better than that?

Up To You

Yet, losing your figure or keeping it is up to you. Some men like reasonably round women, especially as they age and become rounder themselves. They believe such women are more comfortable to live with, and fly from the skinny scarecrows that pose for fashion pictures, calling them "humanoids" devoid of feminine charms. On the other hand, our culture looks down on fatties. They find it harder to get jobs, harder to get clothes, and are snickered at behind their backs.

Probably the best idea is to be content to stay "thin enough," just as it is to be "good-looking enough" or "rich enough." The key word here is "enough." A short time ago I saw a sign in a Madison Avenue, New York, dress shop window that said, "You are never too thin or too rich." Balderdash. They were selling small size, expensive dresses. Keeping extremely thin can become a mania, just as becoming enormously rich can. The happy people are those in the middle ground.

In the final analysis, therefore, it is your decision.

The writer Alexander Woollcott chose to continue to look like a butterball on a diet full of chocolate creams after making the famous remark: "Why is it that most of the good things of life are either illegal, immoral, or fattening?" But later the dancer Ray Bolger, star of the *Wizard of Oz,* who at seventy-six was as trim as he ever was, kept quoting another famous remark: "Ten minutes on the lips, ten years on the hips."

So if you do choose the chocolate-cream life-style, don't blame it on glands. Or the menopause.

11

You Can Keep Your Mind

A group of club women are gathered around an afternoon bridge table. The game is over, and coffee has not yet been served so there is time for leisurely gossip and talk.

The gossip turns first to good news—Mrs. Bright's new baby, Mrs. Beech's remodeled house, Mrs. Rowland's stunning fur coat. It drifts from these to less pleasant topics—Miss Hart's loss of her sister, old Mrs. Carton's bad arthritis, Sarah Yates' "loss of her mind."

When it gets to Sarah Yates, the conversation becomes animated. "Loss of mind" is always a favorite subject. It has drama, conflict, everything a good story should have. What's more, Sarah's trouble came in her late forties as she approached her menopause. This makes it doubly interesting, for the women around the bridge table are in their middle or late forties too. This story hits home.

From Sarah the discussion naturally goes on to other people who "lost their minds" during the menopause. Most of the women seem to have heard about at least one, and the tales become more and more dramatic.

Soon each woman is trying to outdo the others, until a stranger dropping in might think that all woman during their forties go out of their minds.

Well, obviously they don't. You haven't. I haven't. But

hardly anybody remembers the things that don't happen to people. They mainly remember the things that do.

THE CHANCE IS RARE

The facts are these:

The mental illness about which the club women were talking is called involutional melancholia. The words come from "involution," meaning "a turning in," and "melancholia," meaning "sadness or melancholy." Its chief characteristic is a deep despair. The people afflicted with it usually sit and stare apathetically into space, either doing nothing or wringing their hands and tearing their hair.

But involutional melancholia is not to be confused with the mild depression quite a few women suffer during the menopause —one so mild that nobody but they or their families are aware of it.

Let me repeat this so you will remember it clearly: Involutional melancholia, or the popularly called "going out of your mind," is a disease. It is a melancholy so deep and lasting it can go on for months or years. It is also very rare. What many women experience during their changing years is a passing feeling of blueness; then, as the seesaw rebalances, their normal joy in living returns.

Equally important, statistics show no sharp rise in involutional melancholia around the time of the menopause. Women who do succumb at this time do so mainly by coincidence, or as a result of special and individual stresses that could have set them off at other times in their lives. As Dr. Edward Stieglitz put it, "A woman has less chance of going out of her mind during the menopause than she has of having a brick fall off a roof and fracture her skull on the way home from a shopping tour."

Not only are the actual numbers of women who "lose their minds" exaggerated, their stories are exaggerated, too.

Let's take the story of Sarah Yates, the one that made such good conversation. What are the real facts in the case?

Sarah was a big, awkward, homely girl. Her well-to-do parents had never given her much attention, nor had she had much love in her life; she pretended to herself, though, that she was never bothered by any of this.

Rather unexpectedly she married a man who owned a fair-sized Chicago department store. He was so engrossed in making money he didn't have much time or attention left to give Sarah, but since she continued to pretend she didn't expect any, the arrangement seemed to work out. That is, it worked until her only son became engaged. Then suddenly she realized that giving up her son was more than she could bear.

She began to do everything she could to delay the wedding. She insisted, for instance, that she couldn't find a single dress in the whole city that would do for a wedding, not one. How could she let him get married unless she had a proper dress? When her husband produced a smart dress for her, she insisted she couldn't find a proper hall for the reception. When he found a hall, she insisted there wasn't a caterer whose food was fit to eat; and so on.

When finally dress, hall, and caterer had been found to everybody else's satisfaction and the wedding date was set, she tried her last card and threatened suicide. She "had never been a well woman," she said, and now was going through her menopause besides. This marriage would kill her, or she would kill herself.

In the threat of suicide she revealed her true feelings, panic over losing the only person she had ever really loved, or who loved her, plus great hostility to the husband who had not given her the affection she craved. Not only did she threaten she'd kill herself in time to prevent the wedding, she swore she'd do it the week before Christmas. "If I die the week before Christmas, everybody will have to take time off to mourn me," she said. "Then Henry will have to close the store so that the employees can come to my funeral. And won't *that* hurt business right in the middle of the Christmas rush!"

Nobody believed she'd actually try to kill herself. But when she did try, they realized she needed medical help.

At first they took her to a gynecologist in the time-old belief that her troubles were menopausal. The gynecologist referred them to a psychiatrist who placed her in a sanitarium at once.

There, luckily, she found an understanding doctor who let her talk herself out. She began to see a great many things she had never seen before, including the necessity for letting her son go, because only in that way could she keep his love.

Sarah was back home within a few months, not completely remade as a person of course, but well enough so that she could try to make her new daughter-in-law feel welcome. And in the trying many of her own troubles disappeared.

This is the true story of Sarah Yates. As with most stories you hear, either you don't get all the details, or the illness has little or nothing to do with the menopause. Or so many other factors enter in you can't see the forest for the trees.

IT HAPPENS TO SPECIAL TYPES

But even in the few cases where people do go out of their minds, there's another important fact to remember. This is that it happens, as a rule, to certain types of people: rigid people, pleasureless people, and people with dead-end jobs.

Rigid people are the type who can't seem to meet change. The best way to describe them perhaps is with the phrases their friends use about them. Phrases like: "You can set your clock by her, she's always so prompt." Or "She's a fanatic about the house; if her carpet gets one spot on it, she throws a fit." Or "She hasn't changed a thing about herself, not even the way she wears her hair, for twenty years."

Pleasureless people are the type who seem to be always gloomy. Their friends say: "She's only happy when she's worrying." Or "She's always telling about her 'sacrifices' for her family. If there's been nothing to sacrifice, she invents something!" or "She loves nobody, not even herself."

And as for *people whose jobs run out at middle age,* they're the type who find themselves in the prime of life, yet jobless, because their careers were dependent on their youth. Ballet dancers, for instance. Circus performers. Fashion models. Romantic movie stars. Athletes.

Many people with youth-oriented jobs have avoided despair

by doing what Mikhail Baryshnikov did; he became director of the American Ballet Theatre when he knew he had only a few years left in which to dance. Or Beverly Sills, who became director of the New York City Opera when she felt her voice was going. Or Robert Redford, who added movie directing to acting because he knew that soon he might not be able to continue as a romantic star.

On the other hand, there are so-called "Jewish Mothers," women who did not plan ahead. They were so wrapped up in their children that cooking and cleaning for them became an obsession. When these children were ready to go out on their own, these mothers were totally lost.

Dr. Pauline Bart of Indiana University did a special study on "Jewish Mothers" and found a great deal of depression among them. If, for instance, their children married and moved to a home nearby, the mothers demanded a long daily visit; if they moved to a distant town, a long daily phone call. Otherwise they said they had nothing to think about and nothing to plan for, and some even landed in mental hospitals as a result.

Dr. Bart says it is not fair to laugh at such mothers, however, or even to criticize them unduly, because they were only doing what the society they grew up in told them to do. Almost the only time they were praised was when they were bearing and raising a large brood. By using all their energies to bear and raise this brood, it was as if they were "making a deal" with life, one that would give them eternal happiness in return. And when the deal didn't work out they became depressed because they felt cheated and lost.

Today things are different. Today child-bearing and child-raising occupy only a small part of a woman's life. According to our latest figures, the average age of first marriage is twenty-two. A married woman has an average of two children two years apart, and finishes her child-bearing at the age of twenty-six. This means that when her children reach eighteen, or the age at which they become independent of her whether they leave home or not, she is only forty-four. And if she lives to the age of seventy-seven, that means she will have over thirty years left, or a large part of her total life span, with no children to raise.

What is she to do with this large part of her life? Dr. Bart believes she should plan for it in advance, keep her hand in, as it were, in order not to run the risk of becoming totally depressed and lost.

Luckily, few women do become totally depressed. Temporary depression is quite common during the menopause, but ninety-seven percent of all women swing back on their own. Put the other way, the number who suffer from long-term depression is only three percent.

STILL, THERE ARE STORIES

Still there are many stories—too many stories—of women who "go out of their minds" during the menopause. Where do these stories come from? And why have they persisted so long?

The answer is: we probably heard them from our mothers, who heard them from their mothers, who in turn heard them from women who lived long ago.

Things were very different long ago. Many women *did* go insane as a result of drug addiction. According to Ed Brecher's book *Licit and Illicit Drugs,* the eighteenth and nineteenth centuries were "a dope fiend's paradise." Opium, heroin, and cocaine were so freely sold men and women did not even need a prescription for them. They could simply walk into neighborhood stores and buy them, or order them by mail.

A letter from a Philadelphia doctor to a local farmer dated 1781 said, "The opium you sent us was pure and of good quality. I hope you take care of the seed." And during the Civil War years, not only drugstores but grocery stores were selling opium, heroin, and morphine. In Iowa, for instance, a state that had a very small population then, three thousand grocery stores were selling such drugs as casually as they sold sugar or bread.

It was the same in England. Brecher tells about a man who went into a grocery store in London, put a penny down on the counter, and a pillbox full of opium was pushed across the counter without a word being said.

Also, such drugs were freely advertised in newspapers and magazines under attractive names like Mrs. Winslow's Soothing Syrup, Geoffrey's Cordial, or Ayer's Cherry Pectoral. These ads recommended them as "good for woman trouble" or simply called them "women's friends."

The ads were so attractive, indeed, and run in such a variety of papers that all kinds of women, rich and poor, bought them in huge quantities. The poor to quiet their pains and hunger, the rich to relieve their boredom. As a result, many women quickly became addicted, and their families, not knowing what else to do, either looked on indifferently or called them insane.

It wasn't until 1942 that the sale of addictive drugs like heroin, opium, cocaine, and laudanum (laudanum is cocaine dissolved in alcohol, which makes it doubly potent) became illegal in America. But until then, women "went out of their minds" by the thousands, and stories about them spread.

Falling Apart

Becoming seriously ill or depressed is one thing. Falling apart is another. And many women do fall apart during times of stress.

We fall apart, says psychiatrist Dr. Frederic Flach, because we have unreal expectations. We expect all life to proceed the way physical growth does. That is, we know that from babyhood on we will steadily grow taller and taller until, with no effort on our part, one day we will stop. And emotionally we expect the same steady progress.

But emotionally matters are different. Here growth is interrupted by periods of standing still, as well as by periods of confusion or falling apart.

Take, for instance, puberty. During puberty we become confused when menstruation suddenly hits us. (It always seems sudden, no matter how well we have been prepared.) We also are upset when our formerly straight body develops breasts and hips that make us self-conscious, develops feet that fall all over themselves, and a potbelly that sticks out where we had a flat belly before.

Then take adolescence. Now we fall apart with violent mood swings. We feel wildly elated when boys find us attractive, greatly disappointed when they do not. We also get terribly angry at our parents when they disagree with us, deeply hurt by any criticism because it is hard to take.

Then there is the falling apart after marriage. We get engaged in a state of excitement as we look forward to spending our lives with someone we love, to the glamour of the wedding, the beautiful gown we will wear, the flowers, the music, investing all with a romantic glow. But the humdrum chores that follow are far from romantic. Soon there comes the need to cope with money problems, to wash dirty dishes, to pick up after a man who throws his soiled socks under the bed and drops ashes all over the floor.

When such things happen, and some usually do, the time of early marriage can become either a period of standing still, or a time when we feel ready to scream.

Then come pregnancy and birth. Pregnancy can make us fall apart with a vengeance. Because again, no matter how much we have read about pregnancy or been told about it by friends, the great hormonal changes of the first few months come as a surprise and a shock. And during the last few months the problems of waiting and of managing an unwieldy body can be terrific indeed.

And after the "little angel" we dreamed about is born? It can turn out to be the wrong sex, look like the wrong parent, or be not merely an angel but a creature that soils endless diapers, gets hungry at odd hours, wakes up and howls at unexpected times during the night.

And so it goes. Emotionally, we learn, almost never does life proceed steadily upward and onward. We can fall apart again and again.

But the point is, after we fall apart, we can come back together again. Come back, in Dr. Flach's words, "if we have a certain hunger for change; if we are willing to take risks, to be hurt to the point of pain . . . give up something valued and familiar;

accept the feeling of being lost and without bearings until we come back together in one piece."

FIND A JOB

One of the best ways to get over emotional upheavals is to find a job. I must stress this over and over again. As I write this, a little over half of all American women have outside jobs, some because they need the money, some because they enjoy working. Some to replace loneliness and depression with self-esteem. Indeed, from 1900 to 1970 the number of women aged forty-seven to sixty-four who have gone to work has increased by three hundred percent.

Granted, as I said, finding a job if you've been out of the market for a long time is not easy. To be sure, there are problems both practical and psychological.

The chief practical problem is that the jobs offered to you will as a rule pay much lower wages than the same jobs offered men. Also, you are almost sure to find that whatever skills you once had are rusty.

The psychological problems are the difficulty in being assertive enough to talk back to your husband if he insists he's too proud to have you work because a job of yours may diminish his status as a dominant male. This hurdle can be especially difficult if you go into the same field that your husband is in and compete with him; it takes a rare man like a Pierre Curie to work actively with a Marie Curie and keep a happy household. Also, there's the problem of being called "selfish" by your family because you admit to them that for the first time in years you are thinking mainly of yourself and are trying to fulfill yourself as an individual, rather than as a member of a group.

The practical problems? Obviously, if you are offered a lower wage than you think you're worth, you may have to accept it. Also if your skills are rusty, you'll have to brush up on them even before you go out, and that entails hard work.

In his book *Choices,* Dr. Flach has some timely tips to offer: Start thinking of yourself as a new kind of person. Form a dream of yourself as somebody quite different than the woman you now are. You've been seeing yourself mainly as a combination cleaning woman, seamstress, chauffeur, cook, financier, general aide and comforter? Start thinking of yourself as a professional in one particular field that relates to these. You've been making your own or your children's clothes? See yourself as a seamstress to whom people will pay money when you alter or make their clothes. You've been a creative cook? Form a dream of yourself as a restaurant owner, or a caterer who puts together memorable weddings and parties at a price. You find balancing your monthly checkbook easy and pleasant? Picture yourself as an accountant who specializes in doing bookkeeping for small firms.

Next, having pictured yourself as a professional, find out what it takes to become one. If you have seen yourself as an accountant, ask around and discover where up-to-date courses in accounting are being given. A restaurant owner or caterer? Find out where you can study quantity buying and cooking, which is very different from at home. A professional seamstress? Polish up your sewing skills, get a really good sewing machine, on time payments if need be, and practice doing such excellent work that, when you do get customers, they will recommend you to others.

Make sure, however, that your dream is a realistic one. Nine out of ten small businesses—restaurants immediately come to mind—fail after only one year. Becoming a secretary or clerical worker is therefore far more realistic. There is a constant demand for skilled clerical workers and secretaries of all ages. In big cities there are even a few employment agencies that specialize in placing women age fifty-five and older, and some large companies prefer to hire them because they are extremely dependable.

If you are in doubt about your abilities and the practicality of your dream, job counseling is in order.

Finally, sit down and make a list of the friends and relatives who may be able to help you achieve your dream, whatever it is, and then make an appointment to meet them at a place where you can talk freely and frankly. You may be surprised how many ideas friends and relatives can sometimes come up with, ideas that you haven't thought of yourself.

Take the story of Nellie.

Nellie was a red-haired friend of my mother with a homely face and a cheerful smile. The wife of a successful lawyer, she had trod a familiar path all her married life. But when her husband died suddenly, leaving her, to her surprise, with very little money and four children to bring up, she was caught short.

True, she had been a section manager in a large department store before she was married, but that was many years ago. She was in her fifties now, and her terrible feet wouldn't let her do that kind of work. What could she do instead? She had no idea.

She decided the best person to speak to was her husband's brother who was house-doctor at the Metropolitan Opera. She had never talked intimately to him before, but he told her he knew many wealthy singers who did not have either the time or the desire to go shopping; he'd be glad to introduce her to them by letter or phone. Maybe she could tell them she was willing to take fine lingerie samples to them so they could pick out underwear at their leisure. Certainly, he agreed, this would involve walking and taking public transportation, but after she got to the homes of the singers she would almost surely be able to use her cheerful smile and ask them to let her sit for a while and rest.

Nellie asked around again, contacted a wholesale lingerie house, filled a suitcase with samples, and carried them on her terrible feet from one opera singer to another every morning for two years. After that she had enough know-how to open a lingerie shop in her own home, a shop that kept them going in modest comfort until her children began to suppport themselves.

Nellie, in Dr. Flach's words, had that "certain hunger for change," that "certain willingness to take risks." She was able to give up her familiar role of a dependent wife and take on another, until she came back together in one piece.

Displaced Homemakers

But Nellie was a woman of my mother's generation, a generation in which divorce was rare. If her husband had had any money he would have had to leave her, in most states, at least half.

Today the situation is far different. Today the divorce rate is staggering; and to make things worse thirty-one American states have enacted "no-fault" divorce laws, making it possible for a husband or wife to walk out of a marriage for reasons such as incompatibility, meaning the breakdown of the relationship in general, and to do this instead of using adultery as the reason (an "adultery" often cooked-up to convince the court that a divorce was in order).

As I write this, in states where no-fault laws are in force, it is usually the husband who walks out, and if he has no children under eighteen that the law makes him support, the wife is apt to be left stranded. For very few women are awarded alimony on their own. The number who get such an award has been estimated by *Time* magazine to be as low as fourteen percent.

To make things worse, even those women who are awarded alimony seldom collect it, or collect it for long. If a husband moves to another state he often simply stops paying it, and going after him involves hiring a lawyer, something a stranded woman can seldom afford, especially since she may have to do it all over again month after month after month.

Women whose husbands walk out on them are among the group of women called Displaced Homemakers, and they get a jolt because of what happens to them both financially and in terms of their self-esteem. A displaced homemaker has an age range of thirty-five to sixty-five, meaning that she is usually too young to collect Social Security, even if she worked at an outside job before marriage, and too old to quickly get a new job. Nor is she eligible for unemployment insurance because her years of toil inside the home are not considered "work" by the government.

It was a California woman, Tish Sommers, who coined the phrase Displaced Homemakers. Left with almost no funds herself at age fifty-seven when her husband walked out on her, she joined forces with a forty-eight-year-old widow, Laurie Shields, in a similar plight. Together they began to travel around the country and talk to anyone who would listen. Now, largely due to their efforts, there are many Displaced Homemaker Centers, in some instances even funded with government money, with women leaders to run them.

But government money or not, the centers face many problems. Before anything else can be done, says Sommers, a counselor has to help a woman rebuild that shattered self-esteem. She quotes Dr. Jean Baker Miller who reminds us that tradition expects a woman to be the one to keep a marriage going; keep any kind of relationship going, in fact. And since women have gone along with this tradition, as a rule they feel devastated when a relationship fails.

Then, after rebuilding a woman's self-esteem, the leader of a Center takes on the task of convincing the community that a walked-out-on woman is able to hold down a job no matter what her age. And after this, she has to tackle the problems of scouting the area for possible jobs, showing members of the group how to write a résumé, and how to conduct themselves during a job interview after one has been arranged.

None of this, again, is easy.

In areas like Texas where the economy has been booming compared to the rest of the United States, it takes a minimum of persuading to get companies to take in older women. In other places older women often have to start their own businesses like Nellie did, or settle for offbeat jobs like road-crossing guards at schools, announcers at educational television stations, hairdressers at retirement homes.

All in all, job-hunting for an older woman takes courage and imagination. Also a sense of humor. The Oakland, California, Displaced Homemaker Center has this motto hung on its wall: "She who waits for a Knight in Shining Armor will have to clean up after his horse."

It is certainly better whenever possible to get a horse of one's own.

Getting Rid of Anger

All of us have some anger and hostility within us, and we have more of it as we grow older and discover that the world is not quite the warm and comfortable place we imagined it to be.

The best way to get rid of pent-up anger, says the psychiatrist Dr. William Menninger, is by work, outside the home or in.

Lashing out at things instead of people. Lashing out physically by pushing a vacuum cleaner furiously across a floor, shaking a mop, pulling up weeds, kneading bread. Or if for some reason we can't do any of these, taking a long fast walk, or going to the kind of play or movie that will let us have a good long cry.

Surprisingly, a movie that gives us a good cry is better than one that gives a good laugh. The Greek philosopher Aristotle knew this long ago, when he spoke of a drama as a "tragic catharsis" or purge. To him a drama was a play in which there was a hero a little better than ourselves, but not so much better we couldn't identify with him. And since he was better, we felt he didn't deserve the failure the fates handed out to him. We therefore felt terror while he was in the process of failing, and pity when he did. And as we experienced this terror and pity, we cried, and after crying, we left the theater purged of the pent-up emotions that had been too heavy to bear.

Luckily, crying is permitted in women; we can indulge in it freely as long as we can find an approved place, like a theater, in which to cry.

I read an unforgettable short story some years ago about a poor, distracted cleaning woman. Her little nephew, who lived with her, was dying and she could not weep in front of him. It wasn't right for her to weep in her employer's house either, or on the street, and she did not have the money to go to a show. Yet she had to weep somewhere. She finally stumbled into a telephone booth, closed the door and cried herself out there.

But work off tension we must, whether through physical exertion or weeping, because otherwise it can turn back in on ourselves, turn back and cause some of the tension headaches women suffer from, the colitis, the stomach trouble. The popular descriptions of something that makes us angry, "That burns me up!" or "That gives me a pain in my stomach!" are quite literally true.

SAD HOTEL WOMEN

Because of this, there are no sadder women in the world than the rich women who live in luxury hotels. An occasional few pampered weeks in a hotel are fine. But women who live in one indefinitely with no housework to do, no cleaning, no cooking or creative job of any kind, dam up their natural outlets for hostility. This accounts for the eternal shopping sprees in which they dash from one store to another, buying clothes mainly to wear when they go out and buy other clothes, rather than from need. Their savage gambling sprees, or their bridge battles in which everyone bares her fangs.

Hotel women, even more than career women, are the great complainers about insomnia. Dr. Menninger puts this into a memorable sentence when he says, "The trouble with doing nothing is that you cannot rest from it."

Talk

I've talked about work as a great tension-releaser. Talk is another, as we know from the success of consciousness-raising or "rap" groups. For talk is a form of ventilation that releases tension like ventilating a musty room does; after it, the air feels cleaner. Talking with friends is good; talking with a priest, minister, rabbi, or doctor is still better because such people are trained to do a special kind of listening, and are sworn, moreover, not to tell. The Catholic Church has long recognized the value of talk in its use of the confessional, and psychiatrists tell of patients asking each other in wonder, "How did I get better simply by talking to that woman or man?"

So lose your mind? Ninety-seven percent of us won't. Not if we have the courage to fall apart if need be, then pull ourselves together by these many means, and go on again.

12

Is There a Male Change Too?

A few years ago a large number of middle-aged American men started getting the jitters. They ran to drugstores and doctors' offices, pleading for hormones. "We've heard that hormones can do wonders for men as well as women," they cried. "Please, Doctor! Please, Druggist! Don't you think we might try some too?"

This came about largely as the result of a sensational little volume called *The Male Hormone* that had just been published. In it the author, Paul de Kruif, using chapter-headings such as "The Rescue of Broken Men," implied that practically all men around the age of fifty had a "male change" just as their wives did. They suffered not only the flushes, the headaches, the crying spells and the rest, but worse, they suffered an almost total loss of potency. So the picture for the average middle-aged man, at least until he hurried up and took some hormones, looked black indeed.

Well, time has proven him wrong. There almost never is a "male change" in the literal sense of the word. Let's look at the difference between men and women and see why this is so.

THE DIFFERENCE BETWEEN MEN AND WOMEN

A period of changing years, in which her ovaries change their functioning and reproduction stops, is a normal and necessary thing in a woman. It is necessary to protect her from the strain of further childbearing. It is necessary to protect the race by having most babies born to young mothers. It is especially necessary so that mothers can start bringing up their children while they themselves are still young. For bearing children is only a small part of a woman's job. Bringing them up takes much longer—almost twenty years. And when a woman of say forty-five starts to do this, she's sixty-five before she's through. And in the old days, when the great laws of life were laid down, a woman simply didn't live that long.

So a change for a woman is part of nature's plan.

But a man's part in childbearing and child rearing has traditionally been comparatively small. He helps to create the baby, and to a certain extent (although in American society the father's role is changing dramatically) that is that. So nature lets him do his part almost to the end of his days.

As a result, a period of changing years for men, in which their reproductive powers suddenly end, just doesn't seem to be in the cards. Nor does research reveal the presence of any such thing.

According to Dr. Arthur Grollman, professor of experimental medicine at Southwestern Medical College, this happens to as few as one man in a hundred. Others say one in a thousand. And when it does, far from being normal, it's an illness. What is called a "primary testicular failure." A man's male hormones fade out earlier than might be expected, and nobody knows why.

THE DISCOMFORTS ARE SIMILAR

When a testicular failure does occur, however, the physical discomforts may be surprisingly like a woman's. There may be frequency of urination, flushes, fatigue—the list down the line. This is due to the fact that the cause is similar: failing testes, like failing ovaries, cease to balance the pituitary on the gland seesaw.

A doctor I know, a Seattle man, Jim Dunne, suffered such a testicular failure around the age of fifty. A highly regarded specialist in obstetrics and gynecology, he volunteered for service in a Saigon Maternity Hospital during the Vietnam War. Though he was working in an air-conditioned room, he found himself having severe hot flushes as well as a dramatic falling-off in potency. He sent back home for some depo-testosterone (the injectable form), and gave himself a series of injections. After several months of such injections the flushes were gone and his potency was nearly back to what it had been before. "My potency wasn't quite as good," he explained. "But it was satisfactory." Now he is back in the States, remarried, and head of a West Virginia hospital. Everything in his life, he says, is going very well.

But Jim is one of those rare cases. Other men suffer a lessening of potency for purely emotional reasons. Indeed, many doctors feel that a dramatic loss of potency coming early in life is almost never due to purely physical causes. For a man to become impotent because of testicular failure is extremely rare.

Dr. Alfred C. Kinsey's research bears this out. Dr. Kinsey found that instead of a sudden drop, male potency reaches a high in the late teens and early twenties, then shows a slow, steady decline to old age.

In his *Sexual Behavior in the Human Male* he says:

"From the early and middle teens, the decline in sexual activity (of men) is remarkably steady, and there is no point at which old age suddenly enters the picture. . . . There are no calculations in all of the material in human sexuality which give straighter slopes than the data showing the decline with age. . . .

"Even in the most advanced ages, there is no sudden elimination of any large group of individuals from the picture. Each male may reach a point where he is, physically, no longer capable of performance, and where he loses all interest in further activity. But the rate at which males slow up in these last decades does not exceed the rate at which they have been slowing up and dropping out in the previous age groups. This seems astounding, for it is quite contrary to the general conception of aging processes in sex.

"At sixty years of age (only) 5 percent of the males studied were completely inactive sexually. By seventy, nearly 30 percent of them were inactive. From there on, the incidence curve continues to drop. . . .

"Only a portion of the male population ever becomes impotent before death . . ."

Dr. Robert N. Butler of the National Institutes of Health puts this in more specific terms. He says that a man in his teens and early twenties is quick to reach erection, and after an act of intercourse can quickly perform another. A man of sixty, however, is slow to reach erection and must rest for hours before he can perform again. In fact, for reasons we'll come to, he may not be able to perform on occasion for days or weeks. Also, according to Dr. Robert N. Rutherford, a man in his teens and twenties has a stronger sheer physical drive. He desires, and is able to have, an average of 4.5 acts of sexual intercourse a week. A man of fifty an average 1.8 per week; a man of sixty 1.3. But this is strictly average. Every man has to find his own norm, and to realize that this slowing down is natural. Yet because men of fifty and sixty forget that they are no longer teenagers or twenty-year-olds, they often think this falling off is abnormal when it isn't.

And because they think of it as abnormal, some run to doctors pleading for the hormones they hope will restore them to their earlier full capacity. But hormones can't; they may even do just the opposite, because androgen taken from the outside can calm down the pituitary *too* much. When that happens, the pituitary stops stimulating the man's own testes, with the result they become so lazy they make even less androgen than before.

This couldn't be more important for an older man to remember. He may be, say, contemplating a second marriage, and naïvely trusting to androgen to give him a new sexual lease. Instead of a new lease, it may rob him of the one he still has.

Among the few men who take androgen in large quantities are professional weight-lifters. They do this because it is a hormone which helps increase their arm muscles to a tremendous size and strength. But they can take it for only a limited period, and then must slowly taper off, or their pituitary may stop working altogether.

Just as hormone treatment must be carefully supervised for a woman, so, too, must it be for a man. Any man who suspects he has a true testicular failure should see the soundest doctor he can find. Such a doctor will first talk to him at length, asking him about his business, his family, his health in general. For, as with a woman, so many of the "change" symptoms can be confused with other things, or be due to other causes which must be carefully ruled out. Fatigue in a mature man, for instance, can come from a dozen reasons. So can headaches, vague pains, and the rest. While as for that scrap-heap feeling called nervousness—who can easily put his finger on that?

Next, a doctor will take laboratory tests. Tests of a man's urine, or a smear from his penile discharge. He may even perform minor surgery, and put a small piece of his testes under the microscope. There is no room for guesswork here.

If, after all the evidence is in, the doctor decides a course of treatment is in order, it will in all likelihood be testosterone. This will relieve the physical distress, especially distress such as frequency of urination or great and persistent fatigue. Frequency of urination will be relieved because androgen helps the body retain water. Fatigue will be relieved because androgen is a great strength hormone.

However, androgen is no "magic bullet" as Paul de Kruif implied. Since true testicular failure *is* an illness, a man may not find a quick cure. He certainly won't limp into a doctor's office one day and dance out with full potency restored the next.

Of course there are men who bypass a doctor. Some men eat oysters in great quantity, probably because they are soft and round like testicles, and think this gives them a kind of magic power. Others use a mechanical stimulator inserted into the rectum. (The rectum and the genitals are separated by a thin wall, as women in labor who are examined through the rectum know.)

The oysters are harmless. The mechanical stimulator is not; used to excess, it can damage the sensitive rectal tissues.

SOME MEN SHOULDN'T TAKE ANDROGEN IN ANY EVENT

Also, there are some men for whom androgen may be bad medicine in any event. These include men with prostate trouble, men who suffer from a tendency to retain water, and men who hope to father another child.

Men with prostate trouble should take androgen with extreme care because an excess of male hormone may cause dormant prostate trouble to flare up.

If a man is suffering from, say, swollen ankles due to an abnormal water retention, it doesn't make sense to make these ankles swell some more by taking androgen.

And as for men who hope to father another child, this puts a very large question mark before hormone treatment. Many men never give up the hope of fathering another child; at least, it makes them feel proud to know they could have one if they would. And while androgen does increase potency, oddly enough it may decrease fertility. That is, it may lower the sperm count just enough so that a child cannot be conceived.

Now no one understands why the last is true. But extensive research by Drs. Carl G. Heller and William D. Maddock of the University of Oregon Medical School have borne it out. Many men lose their fertility almost completely while taking androgen. In some cases, the fertility returns when the treatment is stopped. In other cases it does not; permanent damage is the result.

ANDROGEN MAY NOT ALWAYS INCREASE POTENCY

Perhaps the greatest joker in the androgen deck is the fact that it doesn't always increase potency. This curious state of affairs may come about because androgen taken as medicine may sometimes calm down the pituitary *too* much. When that happens, the pituitary stops stimulating the man's own testes so that they become lazy and make even less androgen than they were making before.

ANDROGEN MAY ACTUALLY SHORTEN LIFE

And if this weren't enough, androgen taken as medicine may shorten a man's life.

Almost all men ask themselves at one time or another:

"Which do I prefer, a long life or a merry one?" They ask this question because to a certain extent it is up to them to choose.

The men who choose the merry life often drink to excess, smoke to excess, push their sex powers to the limit and beyond. And no one can quarrel with them if their eyes are open and that is what they want to do. But at least they should be aware of the fact that some artificial stimulation of sex activity, pushed by androgen or other means beyond normal limits, can overstrain the heart. For the genitals are only one part of the body. You can't push them harder than the entire body can stand.

Now this is not to say that sex activity suited to a man's age is bad for him. Just the opposite. It can be both enjoyable and a positive good. But overactivity, stimulated by hormones or other means, is something else again.

All in all, a "male change," or true testicular failure, turns out to be a rare illness needing the attention of a skilled physician. Androgen taken for such a true failure can be a boon. Used for other purposes, a doubtful blessing.

13

Love After Forty, Fifty, and Sixty

If there is no such thing as a true and universal male change, why is there sometimes a letdown in a man's potency around the age of fifty just the same? Not a sharp drop, but enough of a letdown so that a formerly loving husband may retreat from marriage-bed to living-room sofa? And why, if this happens, does the woman in the case jump to the conclusion, "He doesn't love me any more?"

There are several answers:

The first is that sex is both an emotional and a physical experience and, as I said a while back, the emotional far outweighs the physical.

Now a man of fifty, give or take a few years, may consciously or unconsciously be going through an emotion upheaval. An upheaval that is sometimes mild, sometimes shattering. For he is often in the process of reappraising his whole past life, and getting ready for the years to come. This upheaval happens to every man. Indeed, as the Yale University psychologist Daniel J. Levinson says, when it is mild it is the mid-life transition; when it is shattering it is the mid-life crisis.

In order to understand this crisis, let's see what has happened before it occurs.

LEVINSON'S SEASONS

We all tend to think that, once adolescence is over, a man's life glides smoothly along. This is not true. It is filled with high peaks and deep valleys, just as childhood is.

Dr. Levinson reached this conclusion in 1978 when he published *The Seasons of a Man's Life,* a landmark book which, for the first time, thoroughly explored the progression of a man's life from age seventeen through forty-five. In it he reported how he and a group of associates had studied forty different men, grouped in four general types—ten novelists, ten executives, ten biologists, ten workers—in the varied stages or "seasons" of their adult lives. He interviewed them over and over during the course of these many years, and found they had remarkably similar periods of adult development. More, all these periods were filled with turbulence, just as childhood is filled with turbulence. In no case did the men just get uneventfully older, as we used to believe they did once adolescence was past.

Indeed, it took a long time simply to go through the first "season," which meant leaving adolescence and starting to enter the adult world. They had to go through a difficult Novice Phase, a phase that in turn was divided into several periods, none of which could be avoided or skipped. And all these periods gave them pain as well as losses and gains.

The Novice Phase

The novice phase is the time from roughly age seventeen to age twenty-two. It is a novice time because during these years a youth is just a "boy-man." He is still a boy because he needs the warmth and support of his family. He is a man because he is beginning to strike out on his own, especially forming a dream about what he'd like his life to be.

Often during the novice phase he gets married, though he seldom is ready for it. But, filled with a youthful sense of wonder and excitement, and curious to find the treasures he is sure life contains, he takes this giant step, only to discover he's only a novice husband and a novice lover, and if he has children, very much of a novice father.

If he finds a job, he discovers he's only a novice worker, too; he may, to his distress, get fired from several jobs he cockily took on, or have to leave before his boss discovers he can't handle them. If he continues his education, he may fail at the goal he first decided on and have to switch. It can add up to an overwhelming period, throwing him into a state of moderate to severe crisis that he is far too young and inexperienced to resolve. Five out of ten of Levinson's workers described the novice phase as a "rock-bottom time" in their lives.

Nevertheless, there are gains in this period as well as losses. The chief gains are the fact the men discovered in themselves the courage to strike out on their own, as well as to realize they had expected too much the first time around.

Entering the Adult World

By around age twenty-three to twenty-eight the novice phase is over. Now a man actually does enter the adult world. But he does not enter into it fully; his life is still too unstable and too incomplete for that. He discovers he needs friends to help him. If he has married, there may be much "togetherness" with his wife; on the other hand, he may find he has chosen the wrong wife, is not certain of his feelings for her, or cannot seem to mesh his marriage with his work. If he has remained a bachelor, he may feel that something is lacking; he has no "center" to his life because his relations with women have been too casual or too stormy. He can't decide whether to get married now and take on the responsibilities that marriage entails, or to leave that step until the age thirty transition which is soon to come.

The Age Thirty Transition

Since every transitional period lasts a few years, the age thirty transition lasts roughly from age twenty-eight to thirty-three.

Levinson calls this time "a remarkable gift and a burden." It is a gift because it gives a man the breathing space he needs before he settles down; it is a burden because he faces the difficult questions: What have I done with my life so far? What do I want to do? What new directions shall I choose to approach closer to my dream?

The thirty-year-old man, says Levinson, "is full of energy, capability and potential." But he is still only a middle adult. If he wants to maintain the marriage he has made, he must perfect his skills as a husband and lover. Become a better sex-partner. Share more intimacy with his wife than he thought possible before, because "Life is becoming more serious, more restrictive, more 'for real.'" He realizes that if he wants to change his life, if there are things in it he doesn't like, or things missing he would like to have, this is the time to make a start; soon it will be too late.

During the age thirty transition, men as a rule use their abundant energy to make changes. The men who take the transition in relative smoothness use their energy to enrich their lives. They start doing social work for their community, going to museums and concerts as well as to ball games, reach out to others as mentors and guides.

On the other hand, those who have painful transitions feel at times that they cannot go on. It is as if they were swimming against heavy tides, or paddling leaky canoes. In such instances Levinson calls it the age thirty crisis rather than the age thirty transition, because it can become a crisis stage indeed.

Some men during a time of crisis abandon their early religious teachings and grope for new ones. Others make drastic job changes. Still others question their sexual identities and take new women into their lives, then restlessly abandon them and regret it. But this is all part of the confusion of their age.

Settling Down

The age thirty transition over, there comes around age thirty-four to forty the settling down period. Levinson refers to it as a period of Boom, or Becoming One's Own Man.

The Boom period, too, contains pain, losses, and gains. Whatever his job, a man tries hard to become his own man by climbing still further up the ladder of success. At home he tries to have his family look up to him and listen to him as a senior, and do this without question. But he experiences pain because he gets contradictory messages both at his job and from his family. If he works for a corporation he is told at one minute: "Work hard, be fearless, and you'll go far." At the next: "Make trouble and you're dead."

At home he is told at one minute: "Become an authority figure to your children," and the next, "Become a friend or pal." If he does try to become a pal it may bring him into conflict with the little boy who is still strong within himself. Make him again feel, consciously or unconsciously, more of a novice boy-man than he has in a long time. As a result he tries quickly to become a senior whom his family obeys unquestioningly, tries to get obedience by any means, and is upset when this fails.

When Margaret Sanger first met H. G. Wells, who later became her lover, she described him in her diary as "a twinkling boy-man," because Wells had dodged the dilemma by ordering his life almost exactly as he pleased.

As an increasingly famous writer, he did not have serious job problems. As a husband and father he ordered his lovely wife to change her name to Jane because to him this was an old-fashioned name that spelled subservience. He did the same with his children, accustoming them to his going away with no notice and no questions asked, staying away for as long as a year, then returning always expecting and getting a welcome. And he was such a stimulating companion when he was at home that the plan worked quite well.

But few men can go their way as easily as Wells did. Some boy-men become sycophants at their jobs during their late thirties, doing anything and everything to be accepted as "nice guys." Others rebel and speak up, then blame any resulting setbacks on their bosses, wives, or colleagues. A few go so far as to call their bosses "tyrants and corrupters," their wives "seducers and witches."

This blaming of their wives, however, is part of a developmental process. According to the writer John Leonard, it is also a safety valve: "One of the many agreeable aspects of heterosexuality," he says, "is the difference, the friction, between men and women. Love is less a perfect understanding than it is a surprised respect." Blaming their wives, then making up with them, is one way of settling down.

HOMOSEXUALS

What about homosexuals who go through the same adult transitions? What happens to them?

They too, it seems, settle down during the age thirty-four to forty transition. Jack Weil, who is gay, is doing just that. As a novice adult and early adult, by choice he held down eight different jobs in eight years and moved a dozen times, calling himself a nomad and leaving his possessions behind him, except a few family heirlooms, when he did move. Now in his middle thirties, for the first time he is returning to one of his earlier jobs, teaching children with severe learning difficulties. He says he is returning because his pupils asked him to; also because they are youngsters to whom he can express the concerned love he would have tried to give to his own children had he had any. He has also bought a small house, and started holding onto all his possessions because they have begun to mean something to him.

Jack Weil illustrates Levinson's belief that a man during his middle thirties and early forties can move on to greater maturity and approach full adulthood. Soon after, however, around age forty-five, he will enter a transition that is in many ways the most important and difficult of all.

The Mid-life Transition

For around age forty-five the man who thought he had settled down is once more rocked on his heels. He quite suddenly (and remember, it always seems sudden) notices that he does not have as much energy as he had. He cannot run the number of miles he used to; cannot play as many sets of tennis; cannot work as many hours a day. He realizes above all that time is running out and that eventually he must die. This last realization can be so startling that some researchers call the time the mid-life explosion.

Peter, a neighbor of mine when I lived in Cambridge, almost exploded when he found himself running down. With his slender and powerful body, until forty-seven he had pretty much thought of himself as inexhaustible. With four sons age twelve to seventeen he wanted to send to college, he had been getting up at five in the morning, having a quick cup of coffee, walking to the university where he taught computer math, setting his computers, feeding and exercising half a dozen horses for friends who paid him to do it, walking home at midmorning for a light breakfast, walking back to class and teaching until midafternoon, walking home again at midafternoon to have a small lunch, going back to the Graduate Research Center to do a special research job for the Army; coming home again in late afternoon to split the heating wood for his house and have the only meal he ate with his family, then going to bed at nine o'clock so he could do it all over the next day.

For several years I had seen him walking back and forth past my house looking cheerful. Then he began to trudge along seemingly exhausted. Concerned, I went out to chat with him one morning and he admitted he *was* exhausted both physically and mentally, and it was plain he had been shocked by the thought.

Also, he had been thinking hard in other directions. Four children were too many these days for a family who wanted to educate them well; maybe he shouldn't have had them. Maybe his wife should go back to being a bank-teller as she had before, or at least become a more efficient manager of the budget at home. Yes, life could come up again with a lot of problems a man thought he had settled once and for all.

But six months later, he had perked up. He had taken on two more special research jobs, if only to prove to himself he could; had added several more horses to those he was caring for, and was again smiling and wearing one of his odd little hats. (He has a passion for hats.) Now he said to me with a grin: "At least I'll never land on welfare!"

Also, one evening he invited me to be his "date" at a church supper at which his wife was serving and washing dishes. When we started back toward home, while she was still in the kitchen, he thought at first we'd have to hurry and get some gas before the stations closed. But when he looked, he discovered the tank was nearly full, and exclaimed, "That's the doing of my blessed wife!"

He had also evidently been working at his marriage relationship, and was moving along there as well.

Many men do this. Says Harvard's Dr. George Valliant: "The mid-life crisis does not appear always to portend decay. It often heralds a new stage, even though it is an explosive, turbulent time."

It is turbulent because many others, like Peter, still face the main task of the mid-life transition, that of reconciling opposing pulls. We are all pulled constantly in opposite directions. Toward becoming tougher or more tender, staying young or growing old, group-minded, or solitary. The greatest pull is between staying young and becoming old.

Young Versus Old

Everyone constantly faces the dilemma of wanting to stay young and at the same time becoming old. It starts as children when we want to hurry and grow up. But when we have grown, we are pleased when someone tries to guess our age and makes us ten years younger, because that seems to keep us young.

For "young," Levinson says, has many delightful meanings. "It represents growth, possibility . . . potential. It is imaged in "the sunrise, the new year, the blossom, the promise, the vision of things to come."

"Old" also has attractive meanings. We talk of the imposing Father Time, the Rock of Ages, the Wise Old Man. And as we swing between the two: we realize that young and old are both good and bad. "We see that to be young is to be lively, giving, heroic, full of possibilities. But it is also to be imperfectly developed, impulsive, lacking in experience. Similarly, the old person (whatever his age) may be seen as powerful, accomplished . . . but also as tyrannical, impotent, reclusive."

So we seek to balance and choose the best qualities of each, with youth often winning out. But as we do this, we are confronted by one of the sad facts about youth. This is that "the (youthful) hero of the fairy tale does not enter into a life of simple, eternal happiness. That the hero is a youth who must die or be transformed as early adulthood comes to an end."

And this confrontation is very difficult in a society where all around us bloom joyous pictures of youth: we gaze at the men of the Marlboro cigarette ads who are eternally strong and heroic as they ride through beautiful country. We revel in the movies of the old West where the scripts written for John Wayne never told about his hard drinking and many broken marriages, only about his "true grit." We glow as Gary Cooper walks down boardwalk streets ever handsome and fearless, never hearing a word breathed about the face-lift that kept him looking as handsome as he was.

Then we seldom learn the real stories of devil-may-care men like Montgomery Clift.

Montgomery Clift, as we see him, was a combination of a straight body, handsome face, and such beautiful brooding eyes they landed him on the cover of *Life* magazine in his mid-twenties as "a new breed of Hollywood male." Soon after, we see him posing jauntily with Elizabeth Taylor who had begged him to marry her after they starred together in *A Place in the Sun,* while other women are seen flocking to him as bees do to flowers. But no one tells us he knew he could marry no one because he was a bisexual, frightened child—a child who crawled into bed with anyone—man, woman, or couple—who would cuddle him and help him get to sleep. We have to read his biography to find how by his mid-thirties, Clift was drinking so heavily that one night after a party at Taylor's house, high in a canyon above Beverly Hills, he was so drunk he had to ask a friend to drive ahead and pilot him down the slope; how he lost his pilot, crashed into a tree, wrecked his car and smashed the right side of his face so badly it seemed hopeless to put it together again; how the doctors nevertheless managed to wire his face together into a semblance of what it had been, though it became an immovable mask. He was in the midst of making a picture when this happened, we learn, and he tried to get out of his contract, but the studio had invested so much money in the film in progress that they refused. The cameramen were told instead to photograph only the better side of his face, and concentrate on his still magnificent eyes.

Now followed what his biographer calls "the longest suicide in Hollywood history." The picture he was making when injured was a failure; so were the two that followed it, the last prophetically named *The Misfits,* starring with him Marilyn Monroe and Clark Gable. He had added drugs to liquor, and Monroe remarked when he arrived on the set with a huge box of assorted pills, "he's in even worse shape than I am." He was found dead in his early forties a few years later, alone, overdosed, and burned out, sprawled face downward on his bed.

Then we know little about the dashing Errol Flynn who also barely made it past forty, spending the last years of his life sailing aimlessly on his yacht with a fifteen-year-old girl, as if he were trying to suck forth from her the youth he no longer had.

Clift and Flynn, when we come to think about it, were the quintessence of Narcissus, the mythical Greek youth who stood transfixed, gazing at his reflection in the water. An early death for them may have been merciful, for like Narcissus, they could never have borne growing old.

Some actors, however, can bear it. Take Mickey Rooney who won fame as Andy Hardy's Boy, then disappeared for a long time as he went through eight disastrous marriages. Yet, fat and bald, Rooney made a stunning comeback in the Broadway musical *Sugar Babies,* singing in an outsized Admiral's hat and fuzzy white wig, dancing in the Macy's Thanksgiving parade, and later interviewed on numerous TV talk shows with a combination of youthful zest and mature conversation. All this at age fifty-nine.

Rooney had, however painful the private process, reconciled the opposing pulls of youth and age.

Tough Versus Tender

Remaining tough versus becoming more tender is another battle a man has to fight at mid-life. This is because from earliest childhood he has, as a rule, been encouraged to become a supermale —to play games that are rough, develop a body that is tough, lick the other boys on his block, or at least threaten to have his father lick them for him.

In adolescence the heroes he hears praised are Marines, wrestlers, or Olympic athletes, while "sissy" traits like tenderness and gentleness are frowned upon.

In early adulthood his heroes change. Now they are business executives, or other people of strong will and great stamina like surgeons, people who "get things done." If he's become a middle executive, he learns to display his business hero-worship by answering the phone with a barking "Tom Withers," an answer that changes to a pleasant "hello" when he finds you're a friend. He explains his bark by saying that if he didn't start this way and it happened to be his boss how else could he prove he was on his toes?

But by his late thirties this need for supermaleness begins to make him exceedingly anxious, especially when he finds he's losing some of his physical powers. Instead of admitting his anxiety, he often overreacts. Has he been trying to be macho before? He will quiet his fears and become more macho than ever. Try his best to become a daring parachute-jumper who doesn't whine if he is hurt. Or a tight-lipped stock-car driver—a man who under any circumstances will stay in a race beyond his strength.

Sometimes he cannot even allow himself to drop his supermale mask at home and develop a better intimacy with his wife or children, for fear this, too, will emasculate him. As for working under a woman superior—this is something he finds very hard to do.

A CHANGE

But during the mid-life transition there's a change. If he makes a good transition he realizes how foolishly he has been acting and permits himself to become a more tender lover, a more companionable father, a less dominant office boss. He does this because he comes to see that tenderness and compassion have all along been parts of himself, just as have female and male hormones—parts to be proud of rather than ashamed.

Group-minded or Alone

People need people; they need to feel part of a group. They need people with whom they can do business, go to parties or the movies, make social phone calls.

But there is such a thing as compulsive party-going, or compulsive social telephoning. It leaves a man or woman no time in which to meditate, to make long-term plans, to heal from the bustle and flurry of crowds.

During mid-life a man who makes a smooth transition balances his pulls here, too. The Good Time Charlie calms down and spends more time with his family and his community doing worthwhile things. He also discovers the deep feeling of goodness his own company can bring. When Ernest Hemingway wrote his famous story about Nick Adams, the fisherman, he called it *The Big Two-Hearted River*. One heart was the flowing stream; the other the contentment in the heart of the man who was fishing alone.

A man also becomes less competitive, less argumentative, less in need of praise. In Levinson's words: "A man in early adulthood is full of intense desires: to win, to be right, to achieve the noble Dream, to be highly regarded by those that matter (or perhaps, without admitting it, by everyone). With further development in middle adulthood, some of these desires fade away. Those that remain have a less urgent finality. They can also be realized more fully. He can be at the same time more loving and sensual, more authoritative, more intimate, and more solitary . . . Yet he will always waver, sometimes be too attached, sometimes too separate. He will remain a bundle of contradictions, and it is with these he must make his peace."

None of this balancing of opposing pulls is easy; it takes a lot out of a man. As he reviews his past and looks hard at his future, he cannot help but experience a great deal of turmoil. He does so because he has to admit to himself that in all probability he has not, and most likely will not, reach the fullness of his dream. If he's a novelist, he will probably not write the Great American Novel; a scientist, not win the Nobel Prize; a businessman, not become the head of his company. He may write a "good enough" book perhaps; make a reasonably exciting scientific discovery; get to be vice-president of his firm rather than chairman of the board. Beyond that, however, the chances are slim that he will superachieve.

Admitting this to himself is shattering, mildly shattering to some men, deeply to others. And because a man is going through a shattering experience, he may be irrational at times, so irrational he may seem "sick." But he is not so much sick as exhausted (as exhausted as his wife is if she is going through a difficult menopause). Indeed, Alan, a middle-aged businessman, felt so exhausted he stopped me on the street one day and asked, "Is the menopause catching?" His wife was going through a difficult menopause. He was sure he was too. I told him no; it wasn't catching. He was going through the struggle of his own transition. He has gone through many from early adulthood on; he would come out at the other end of the tunnel just as his wife would come out. If he took a deep breath and faced this, he could go on.

Havoc in His Sex Life

Meanwhile, as every man makes an effort to rebalance, the struggle can wreak havoc with his sex life.

Levinson says that a man at mid-life has plenty of energy for a rich and satisfying sex life. That is, he has plenty if he gives up his fantasy dreams about sex and accepts "good enough" expectations instead of those that are unreal.

Dr. Bernie Zilbergeld, head of the Men's Training Program of the Human Sexuality Program of the University of California in San Francisco, speaks about these unreal expectations.

Most grown men, he says, have fantasy expectations about sex that date back to the time when they were boys. Boys around thirteen start to do a lot of thinking about sex because the male hormones that flood their bodies give them strong sexual feelings. But they know almost nothing about the subject except that somehow, in some way, they must "prove" themselves with girls. How to prove themselves? They don't know that either and there's almost no place where they can get information. It's not a subject a boy talks about with his parents as a rule; and if he talks to his friends they know as little as he does, so they either lie or brag. As a result he gets what information he can from books.

Unfortunately, many of the books from which young boys get their information are what Dr. Zilbergeld calls "fantasy books." Books like those written by Harold Robbins and Mario Puzo, which are designed to titillate rather than educate, and do this by taking him into a sexual fantasy land.

Here, for instance, are a few paragraphs from a book by Harold Robbins called *The Betsy,* which, as Dr. Zilbergeld reminds us, is not pornographic in the strict sense of the word, but a book that can be freely and cheaply purchased in drugstores and supermarkets everywhere.

Here Robbins, one of the best-selling authors of fiction in the world, is describing a sex-encounter:

"Gently her fingers opened his union suit and he sprang out at her like an angry lion from a cage . . . Naked, he looked even more like an animal than before. Shoulders, chest and belly covered with hair out of which sprung the massive erection. She almost fainted looking down at him. Slowly he began to lower her down on him . . . It was as if a giant of white hot steel were penetrating her vitals. She began to moan as it opened her and climbed higher into her body, past her womb, past her stomach, under her heart, up into her throat. She was panting like a bitch in heat.

"And finally when orgasm after orgasm had racked her body like a searing sheet of flame and she could bear no more she cried out to him in French.

"'Take your pleasure with me . . . Quick, before I die.'"

Let's take a closer look at this scene:

In the first place, the man's penis is not content to stay in the woman's vagina; it "goes up through her womb, into her stomach, her heart and into her throat," all of which is physically impossible.

Second, it pictures the man's penis as "a giant of white hot steel," another impossibility. The male genital is made of soft flesh, not hard steel.

Third, the woman in the scene has an endless series of orgasms, each not the simple nervous explosion which a female orgasm usually is, but "searing sheets of flame."

Taken together, these paragraphs are so divorced from reality they would be laughable if the boy reading them didn't take them for gospel truth.

In a similar scene from *The Godfather,* the penis is "an enormous, blood-gorged pole of muscle," which, too, is totally unreal. The penis is no more a muscle then it is a piece of steel. But that doesn't seem to bother Mario Puzo, author of *The Godfather,* since his aim is also to excite rather than to educate, and he knows that millions of people will devour his works.

Dr. Zilbergeld examines other fantasy-land penises. He says, "Not only are they larger than life, they also behave peculiarly. They are forever 'pulsating,' 'throbbing,' and 'leaping about.' The mere touch or sight of a woman is sufficient to set the penis jumping, and whenever a man's fly is unzipped his penis leaps out." He gives another example of Harold Robbins', this one from *The Inheritors:* "She pulled open the buttons on his trousers. He sprang swollen into her hand."

Nowhere, says Dr. Zilbergeld with a touch of humor, does a penis "merely mosey around for a look at what's happening" first. It leaps. It springs. This is fantasy land indeed!

But since sex is a subject so seldom honestly talked about, not only does a boy believe these tales, even a middle-aged man continues to do so. He compares his real penis to the models and finds it woefully lacking. Indeed, most men are sure their penises are not what they ought to be. A recent magazine survey of over a thousand men, quoted by Dr. Zilbergeld, found that "all male respondents, with the exception of the most extraordinarily endowed, expressed doubts about their own sexuality based on their penile size. . . . Given what we learned, this isn't surprising. The problem is that we think we should measure up to what are basically impossible standards. The penises in the model are products of fantasy and the real always loses when compared to the creations of human imagination."

PERFORMANCE GOALS

Even worse than doubts about the adequacy of his penis size, an older man has false expectations about his sexual performance, expectations so false they can be devastating to his self-esteem. If he couldn't live up to unreal performance goals at age twenty when he was at the height of his potency, how can he expect to do so at forty-five when his potency has declined?

Also a man at mid-life not only has unrealistic expectations about what he's supposed to be able to do, but unrealistic expectations of what his partners *expect* him to do. Dr. Zilbergeld here criticizes the statements of Masters and Johnson that say about half of women have an unlimited number of orgasms, because the authors don't make it clear that these women had such orgasms through manual self- or partner-stimulation, not necessarily intercourse.

Zilbergeld also criticizes the book *Passages* by Gail Sheehy in which she speaks of "ascending chains of female orgasms leading to ecstasy." Sheehy, he says, makes this sound like a normal occurrence when actually it is extremely rare.

Dr. Wardell B. Pomeroy, one of the original Kinsey researchers and now a California therapist, agrees: "Many women today expect more out of sex, including orgasm and multiple orgasm. One of the problems we have in sex therapy is to try and make these expectations more realistic. For example: if a woman who has never had an orgasm, when asked what she expects it to be like, says that she expects stars to explode and bells to ring, I point out it simply *isn't* that earth shaking. Lower expectations make it easier for her to achieve what she has been seeking."

More Fantasy Books

There are still other fantasy books by writers like the anonymous authors of *The Sensuous Woman* and *The Sensuous Man*. Again these make unreal promises, so that reading them can lead to feelings of great failure on the part of basically healthy men and women when they find they simply cannot live up to what has been described.

Dr. Zilbergeld sums up the situation by saying: "Any fantasy is fine as long as you are aware it's a fantasy and so long as you don't feel inadequate when reality does not conform to it." But, he goes on, society as a whole refuses to give people meaningful and realistic sexual scripts to follow. Most people are so insecure and anxious about sex they believe anything they hear.

As an example, for a time there was a whiskey with the brand name of Kinsey which men drank in great quantities in an effort to increase their potency, because Alfred Kinsey, who had nothing to do with it, had written about sex. But actually liquor is only a stimulant for a short time, then it becomes a depressant, and a man who has drunk too much soon finds he can't have sex at all.

The answer, say the authorities who truly want to help men, is for them slowly, painfully, to work out meaningful scripts of their own tailored to their age and personalities.

Working Out One's Own Scripts

How to work out these scripts?

The first thing to do, write Dr. Robert N. Butler of the National Institutes of Health and his co-author, social worker Myrna I. Lewis, in their book *Sex After Sixty,* is to remember that older men and women are still definitely interested in sex though usually afraid to admit it for fear they will be laughed at, called "dirty old men," "old fools," or "old goats."

"Lustiness in young men," says Dr. Butler, "is sneered at as lechery in older men. Flirtatiousness in young women is put down as depravity in older women."

This kind of talk, he goes on, is grossly unfair. It has been perpetuated by young people who cannot bear to think of their parents as sexual beings, and have gone on to extend their beliefs to older people everywhere. And since nobody seriously asked their parents, the myths grew and grew.

DIFFERENCES IN OLDER MEN

There are, to be sure, differences in sexuality between older and younger men. Dr. Butler spells out these differences and gives us some of the meaningful scripts men have been seeking.

"Most men begin to worry secretly about sexual aging some time in their thirties, when they compare their present level of sexual performance with the level of teenagers and very young adults. These worries tend to accelerate in the forties and fifties and reach a peak in the sixties as definite sexual changes continue to be observed.

"What changes do men notice? Quite simply, their penises don't work as they did at a young age . . .

"The older man ordinarily takes longer to obtain an erection than a younger man. The difference is a matter of minutes after sexual stimulation rather than a few seconds. The erection may also not be quite as large, straight and hard as in previous years. Once the man is fully excited, however, his erection will usually be sturdy and reliable, particularly if this was the pattern in earlier life.

"Premature ejaculation, which is psychologically induced, does not tend to develop for the first time in the later years. It is a symptom that evolves in the earlier years but may continue into later life. Fortunately it is subject to treatment. In addition, premature ejaculation may become less of a problem as a man grows older simply because some of the urgency to ejaculate diminishes.

"Also the lubrication that appears prior to ejaculation . . . becomes reduced or disappears completely as men age, but this has little effect on sexual performance. There is also a reduction in the volume of seminal fluid, and this results in a decrease in the need to ejaculate. Younger men produce three to five milliliters of semen (about one teaspoon) every twenty-four hours, while men past fifty produce two to three milliliters, or about half. Actually, this can be a decided advantage in lovemaking since it means that the older man can delay ejaculation more easily and thus make love longer, extending his own enjoyment and enhancing the possibility of orgasm for his partner.

"Then orgasms may begin to feel different with age. The younger man is aware of a few pleasurable seconds, just before ejaculation, when he can no longer control himself. As ejaculation occurs, powerful contractions are felt and the semen spurts with a force which can carry it one to two feet from the tip of the penis. With an older man there may be a briefer period of awareness before ejaculation or no such period at all. The orgasm itself is generally less explosive, in that semen is propelled a shorter distance and contractions are less forceful. *None* of these physiological changes interfere with the aging man's experiencing extreme orgasmic pleasure.

"Whereas younger men can usually have another erection in a matter of minutes after orgasm, the older man must wait a longer period of time from many hours up to several days, before a full erection is again possible. In addition, in contrast to a younger man's pattern of minutes or even hours in losing his erection, the older man rapidly loses his following orgasm, often so quickly that the penis literally slips out of the vagina. This is not a sign of impairment of the penis and its erectile capacity.

"Older men need not fall into the common trap of measuring manhood by the frequency with which they can carry intercourse through to ejaculation. Some men over sixty are physically satisfied with one or two ejaculations per week because of the decrease of semen production. Others, particularly if they were sexually less active earlier in life, do not ejaculate this frequently. Whatever the customary frequency, and although they can often force themselves to ejaculate more often, if left to choice each man finds his own level. Remember that love-making need not be limited to ejaculatory ability.

"In addition, a pattern of regular sexual activity helps preserve sexual functioning."

Dr. Butler tells of an instance where an eighty-eight-year-old husband and his ninety-year-old wife were regularly making love.

A GOOD AGE

Alex Comfort, author of the well-known *Joy of Sex,* has also
written a book on older people called *A Good Age.* In it he has
this to say: "The capacity for erection is *never* lost through age.
It can become impaired by performance, anxiety, by medication,
by alcohol, by obesity, by diabetes, or by thinking it should be
impaired. The only age changes are in the angle of the erect
penis, which points down while in muscular youth it pointed up,
and in the amount and character of stimulation needed to produce it. In early life [a man] often gets psychic erections [from
thinking about sex or seeing a sexual object] whereas after age
fifty this gets rarer [except in sleep]. Erection may also require
two or three minutes of direct stimulation, by rubbing or otherwise, to bring it about. Both men and women need to know this.

"The rules are: don't worry, don't hurry . . . The com-
monest cause of sexual nonfunction at all ages is performance
anxiety."

And speaking about men who are afraid to resume sex after
a heart attack or other serious illness, Comfort says: "Sex is a
highly undangerous activity. Stopping it unwillingly is far more
dangerous to health than a little exertion; in some people stopping
leads to severe depression. Accordingly, abstinence from sex because of conditions such as a coronary or a major illness should
be limited only to the time when you have actually to abstain
from walking around the room. An old person who has an operation is got out of bed as soon as he or she recovers from the anesthetic, because bed rest in itself causes loss of function. This is
equally true of male sexual function—one real age change is that
if you drop your regular sexual activity for any length of time,
you may have difficulty and need treatment to restart.

"This disuse effect is often seen in widowers, when the wife
dies after a long illness and the man wishes to remarry; here the
disuse, the strange partner and probably some guilt at the relief
natural when a lingering illness ends, can result in difficulty in
getting an erection. In this case get help—the impotency is re-
versible by treatment. You need to defend your sexuality against

both disuse and the assaults of injudicious treatment and advice —for this purpose you need a doctor with whom it can be discussed and who considers your wishes normal. Usually a doctor who fully values his own sexuality will value yours."

It cannot be stressed often enough that men with sex problems are mainly healthy men, not neurotic men. And this applies to young men as well as older men. *Psychology Today* did a survey of fifty-two thousand men of all ages. Fifty-five percent said they were dissatisfied with their sex lives.

Probably this is because much has been written about female sexuality, but less has been written about male sexuality. To repeat: men don't talk to each other, and when they do they are apt to lie. So men get all kinds of mixed up ideas or no ideas. Many unmarried young men don't know how to start a sex life; some even don't know how to approach a woman. While some married men think of sex as a "duty" toward their wives, afraid that if they don't give them what they think they want, someone else will.

The result is a haunting discontent or feeling of failure. Says Dr. Zilbergeld: "The badge of manhood can be worn only temporarily; it can be questioned or taken away at any time. One act poorly done, one failure, one sign of weakness, that's all it takes to lose your membership in the charmed circle. Many men can remember how their teachers, coaches, and friends used this knowledge to keep them in line."

Dr. Jean Baker Miller adds her analysis: "Feelings of weakness, vulnerability, helplessness, are common to all men and women. Such feelings are unpleasant and terrifying, especially to men, who have been taught not to admit they have them. The first step then, is to admit weakness. The next is to add: I feel weak now, but I intend to move on from *that*. Everyone repeatedly has to break through to a new vision if he or she is to keep living on."

What Women Want

What is it that women want sexually from men during the midlife transition? Until now, few men have asked women because sexuality has been defined by men without consulting women. But Dr. Zilbergeld and other well-known researchers have begun to consult them, and the answers are now coming out. When Dr. Zilbergeld, working with a woman, Lynn Stanton, sent out a questionnaire asking women how they felt about sex relations, four hundred replied.

These were their main findings:

First, women want more from men, but "what they want has nothing to do with bigger penises, harder or more frequent erections, perfect performances, or mind-blowing orgasms. They want more of the kinds of things many men are now realizing that they want to give—equal treatment, understanding, sensitivity, communication. Another way of saying the same thing: women want more of what men have not been allowed to give because of the rigid ordering of human qualities into male and female categories. They want men to be more fully human, more fully themselves, so that women can be who they are."

Second, women complain that men do not give enough of themselves, and it is this that often makes them angry and inhibited in bed. Dr. Zilbergeld gives a typical reply:

"He says he loves me but you'd never know it from the way he acts. We never do any touching, talking, or anything else. He doesn't have time for me because he's so busy with all the important things like his job, working on his stupid boat, paying bills and caring for the lawn, and watching a zillion football games on TV. I want more of him. I don't care if the lawn never gets mowed."

Then women want to touch and be touched without relation to sex: "Affection is what I crave. Touching is important all the time."

As to orgasms: Unlike men, who expect an orgasm every time, women say they don't think them particularly important. "I don't want to feel that I have to climax every time. I want to be able to get what I need to have an orgasm when I want one, but that isn't every time I have sex. I want to be able to enjoy just doing what feels good, without worrying how it should end."

And: "If I haven't climaxed but feel warm and happy and sleepy and tell my partner I want to sleep, it makes me angry if he insists I must have an orgasm. That says, 'I'm meeting my male ego needs and to hell with you.'"

Also, women want men to talk. "I like for men to tell me what feels good to them and what they like for me to do sexually. It not only helps me to know what to do but also makes it easier for me to tell them what I like."

The last statement is perhaps the key issue—the fact that women want men to talk to them, and in turn want to talk to men. It is also the most difficult thing for older men and women to do, if only because they have almost never done it before.

However, it is even more difficult for men to talk than for women. Says Dr. Zilbergeld, "It is so difficult it may need advance planning. Planning just what to say and when to say it. And trying again if at the last minute you 'chicken out.'"

A simple sentence with which to start is: "Where do you like to be touched?" It is the sentence Jane Fonda and Jon Voight asked each other in the movie *Coming Home*. Another piece of dialogue in that movie which affected me deeply was when Fonda asked afterward: "Will we always be friends?" and he answered "Always." For if sex is to have any meaning, lovers have to remain friends above everything else.

So speak out when you hear people put down sex and friendship between older men and women. Tell them that they, too, will be old some day, and if the chain isn't broken they will suffer for their careless words. Remind them that sex is good at any age between people who truly love each other. That women never grow old sexually, and men only a little and slowly. And that as one woman describes it, sex in later years is "a warm shelter against the night."

Tell them that Dr. Pomeroy believes it is also a myth that "liberated women" are causing a lot of potency problems in men these days. He insists "there is no data to substantiate this. Women who cause impotence are not truly relaxed and secure about their own sexuality." Helping them to be secure, he believes, is the answer.

From a different source comes cheerful news about older women and happiness in general. This news is that women in their mid-fifties and over are the happiest of any group in America.

Redbook magazine found this out after questioning fifty-two thousand readers on the subject. Rather to their surprise, women in their mid-fifties reported being happier than twenty-year-olds. There was a low period in the late forties and early fifties when a number of women were having menopausal troubles, or difficulties finding new jobs. But after that women spoke of their "great pride in overcoming their feelings of dependency on other people's approval. . . . and a new tolerance and satisfaction with their mates." Gail Sheehy, who analyzed the replies for *Redbook,* sums them up: "Those who take risks turn out to be among the most contented.

"The enlightenment young women can take from this study," she continues, "is that each stage ahead holds the promise of a new beginning in which it is possible to throw off old fears and conflicts, leave behind outlived roles, and release a more certain, valid self who is capable of loving more richly and loving more fiercely."

Loving more richly and loving more fiercely! Could anything bring greater happiness than that?

LEVINSON AND EINSTEIN

Levinson, with whom we started this chapter, deserves a repeat: "Men during mid-life and after have plenty of energy left for a full and satisfying sex life."

To prove it—if it needs proving—here's a story about Albert Einstein told by a woman who knew him well:

"Although it is common knowledge that Einstein had been twice married before he came to the United States, I have never heard a reference to any later romantic attachments. It would seem strange that such a vigorous and warm-hearted man should be totally celibate in his early sixties. In fact, I was a happy and guilty witness to the fact that there was at least one woman in his Princeton life.

"During those years of the early forties, a handsome lady

around forty or fifty with copper-colored hair occasionally visited the Einsteins, and we saw her in the company of the whole family. One evening a friend and I returned to my house after a movie. As we were putting our bicycles in my garage, the light went on in the huge window of Dr. Einstein's studio, which overlooked his back garden. We looked up to see Dr. Einstein and the copper-haired lady standing by the desk. Suddenly, before our incredulous eyes, they fell into a passionate embrace. We were fascinated, horrified, and terribly guilty over our inadvertent voyeurism. At last it proved too much for our girlish consciences, and, giggling desperately, we shone our flashlights into the lovers' eyes. They blinked, started apart, hastily turned out the light and went into another room. I have always regretted disturbing such a happy scene."

There you are again. A man and woman living fiercely and loving richly as life goes on.

And think how much finer a world it would be if men and women understood each other more, and talked to each other more, on such a vital subject as sex.

14

The Estrogen-Cancer Scare

There are many important chapters in this book. In some ways this one is the most important. It talks about the relationship of estrogen to cancer, a subject so controversial, and with such strong opinions on either side, that both women and doctors hardly know where they stand.

The first thing to remember is that for years estrogen was more or less considered a cure-all not only for menopausal troubles, but also for energy loss in the years beyond that. In fact, many doctors saw no reason why they shouldn't give hormones freely until their patients reached the age of ninety, and many patients saw no reason why they shouldn't take them. Other doctors freely prescribed pills containing estrogen for menstrual pain, and also continued giving them for many years.

Then the tide turned. Suddenly estrogen became linked to cancer, with the result that some women refused to take it even when their doctors prescribed it. My sister Helen is an example. Helen had a terrible back and badly needed hormones as a possible preventive of osteoporosis. Yet even though her back got worse and worse she tore up estrogen prescriptions as soon as she left the doctor's office, and by the time she was in her seventies she was barely able to walk.

Then there is Laurie, the daughter of a friend of mine. Laurie had very painful menstrual cramps that a brand of birth-control pill almost completely relieved. But after she got scared she refused to take the Pill, too, and switched to motrin instead.

What happened? How did this turn of the tide come about? First, let's go back to the year 1940.

In 1940, Dr. Lipschutz published a dramatic article in the prestigious British medical journal, *Lancet,* that told of an experiment he had done: for six months he had rubbed the breasts of mice with estrogen and they had gotten the dread disease of breast cancer as a result. The article was researched and written in such detail that it became another of those shots heard around the world.

But what most women and doctors who heard about the article did not know, was that the mice used in the experiment were a special strain, which had been inbred for many generations to produce breast cancer. That is, if allowed to live out their natural lives under the best of conditions, these mice would have gotten breast cancer in any event. Also Dr. Lipschutz had given them doses of estrogen thousands of times stronger than any that could possibly be given to humans. They had been given as much as one thousand milligrams every week for those six months, that is, half their body weight in estrogen for a full fourth of their lives.

Commenting on this experiment, Dr. William Bickers, former professor of obstetrics and gynecology of the American University in Beirut, Lebanon, and now practicing in Richmond, Virginia, says: "It is quite impossible to administer a comparable dose to women. The attempt to translate this mice experiment to women is therefore ludicrous."

What is more, similar experiments were later done with animals closer to people. Monkeys were given estrogen for as long as ten years, but though they got as much as a million rat units a year, no malignant growths occurred. And when this last was publicized many doctors began freely to prescribe estrogen again.

But in October 1975, a new scare started that made some doctors change their minds yet once more. Another article was published in the *New England Journal of Medicine,* which is comparable in prestige to the British *Lancet.* Here two California studies were reported, one done by Dr. Donald C. Smith and associates, and the other by Drs. Harry K. Ziel and William D. Finckle. This said that women who took estrogens had a significantly increased risk of getting cancer of the endometrium (lining of the womb) over those who did not.

The scary words were "significantly increased risk." They were so scary that the Food and Drug Administration immediately took action, announcing that it was planning an insert to be put in every package of estrogen restricting its use to women with hot flushes only. Also, a lower dose should be used than formerly recommended, and the medication occasionally stopped to determine whether or not it should go on.

This announcement of the planned package insert was not made publicly, however. It was made in a closed session of the obstetrics and gynecology committee of the FDA, at which only fifteen members were present. At once sharp disagreements arose between these fifteen members because while some were greatly impressed by the California studies, others were not.

Dr. Douglas Shanklin of the Chicago Lying-in Hospital criticized the California studies by saying he had done studies that proved just the opposite. And a New York doctor insisted that estrogens are not inherently cancer-causing because they cannot cause changes in cells. They can cause growth of cells, to be sure, but the potential for growth depends on the condition of the woman receiving the treatment. Women who seem most prone to cell growth are generally overweight, approaching old age, or have never had a child.

The case against estrogen was far from open and shut.

The discussion at the closed meeting had stirred up so much controversy, however, and the subject was so serious, that an open meeting which drew standing-room-only crowds, soon followed.

At this meeting Dr. Robert Kistner of Harvard University criticized the article in the *New England Journal of Medicine* when he declared that "the microscopic sections in the original California papers had not been reviewed by authoritative gynecologic pathologists prior to publication." He also insisted that the cautions in the proposed FDA package insert were nothing new, but a part of standard medical practice. And Seattle's Dr. Noel S. Weiss retorted in the FDA's defense that "unfortunately many patients are not treated by Dr. Kistner."

And so the controversy grew. It grew so fast that in May 1976, or only a few months after it all started, the medical journal *Current Prescribing* hastened to get out a special report called "The Estrogen Cancer Flap: What You Need to Know." This special report started by telling how Dr. Robert Greenblatt, professor emeritus of endocrinology at the Medical College of Georgia, was receiving several calls a day about estrogen from distressed women and doctors, some women going so far as to declare they were canceling their appointments and "trying to do without." It went on to tell how Dr. Greenblatt had said in reply to the calls that in his opinion the article in the *New England Journal of Medicine* was "sensational" and "extravagant."

On the other side, the special report quoted Dr. Donald C. Smith, who defended the article and recommended a conservative approach. That is, giving estrogen for vasomotor symptoms and atrophic vaginitis (dry vagina) only, since hormones were "extremely effective and beneficial for these conditions." But the key point was to keep dosages low: "I seldom have to exceed 0.3 mg. (a quarter dose) of conjugated estrogens for any of my patients," said Dr. Smith.

Dr. Greenblatt now came on again with a conservative suggestion of his own. He suggested giving patients who need it three weeks of a low-dose estrogen followed by a week of oral progesterone. The purpose of the progesterone was to bring on a bleeding period like a menstrual period, or to shed the endometrium and wash out any possible cancerous cells. Dr. Greenblatt, one of the pioneers in hormone therapy, had already been doing this successfully for twenty-five years.

Current Prescribing's report to doctors ended with a summary of these suggestions, including the journal's own advice, which follows:

- Use the lowest effective doses possible.
- Consider using progestogen (a form of progesterone) during the patient's cycle-off week since some studies suggest that progestogen has a protective effect.
- Immediately investigate . . . all bleeding in non-progestogen

treated patients, and unusual bleeding in patients who are
treated with progestogen.

- Inform patients that there may be some cause for concern,
  and that you are being especially watchful . . . You might add
  that published studies disagree about the seriousness of the disease they associate with estrogen use, and that, when detected
  early, cancer is readily treatable. Further study is urgently
  needed—and that's one thing that everyone agrees about.

But the matter was too important to rest at that. Six months
later in October 1976, the *Medical World News* ran its own discussion on the controversy because, as it said, "Newspapers and
articles in the lay press have heightened the dilemma for women
and their physicians. The answers lie just around the corner. The
American College of Ob/Gyn has been besieged with requests for
its technical bulletins on the subject, which won't be available
until next month. FDA labeling changes, proposed early this
year, still haven't been released . . . Meanwhile the debate continues."

As to diagnosis, the original California studies were again
criticized as inconclusive by the *Medical World News*. It quoted
several doctors who had not been heard from before.

Dr. Betty Ruth Speir, assistant professor of Ob/Gyn at the
University of South Alabama, said she regularly prescribed estrogen for her menopausal patients and expected to use it herself
someday. Yes, the possibility of increased risks bothered her, but
until these were proved she felt the "quality of life" estrogen
allows makes it well worth using.

As to progesterone, the *Medical World News* quoted California's Dr. Howard Judd as saying, "Most of us don't give progesterone now. We are beginning to wonder if we should." And New
York University's associate professor of Ob/Gyn Lila E. Nach-
tigall, insisted that she swore by progesterone. "I've always
believed proliferating (fast growing) endometrial tissue isn't
healthy, and I honestly wouldn't prescribe post-menopausal estrogen without progesterone."

Still, nobody had heard from a psychiatrist. So Dorothea

Kerr, assistant professor of psychiatry at Cornell University, was interviewed by *Modern Medicine* in March 1977.

Dr. Kerr made the thoughtful comment: "I add my concern over cancer phobia. Public discussion of controversies in medical research is causing fear to the point of panic. Such fear may be a necessary by-product in the education of the public so that patients can become informed, cooperative participants, but disabling fear also can turn people away from any examination or treatments."

Now *The Reader's Digest* decided it was time for them to get into the act. So in November 1978 it ran a long article on the subject.

This article was a question-and-answer interview with the internationally recognized endocrinologist and gynecologist Dr. S. Georgeanna Jones, former professor of Ob/Gyn at Johns Hopkins Medical School, and now occupying a similar position at Eastern Virginia Medical School. The *Digest* said the article was triggered by the fact that in September 1977, the FDA had finally prepared two package-inserts, one for estrogen used in menopause, another for the Pill, and ordered them put into every prescription filled in the United States. But—and this was the confusing part—the FDA had not considered estrogen dangerous enough to remove it from the market, as it had done with thalidomide, for instance.

I reproduce *The Reader's Digest* questions as asked by Walter S. Ross and answered by Dr. Jones, some repeating for the sake of emphasis what has been said in previous chapters:

Q. What is the connection between estrogens and menopause?
A. During menopause a woman's body produces less and less estrogens. It's a normal process and does not necessarily have to be treated. But in about 20 to 40 percent of women it produces symptoms severe enough to be unbearable.

Q. What are those symptoms?
A. There are acute symptoms, and delayed ones. The worst acute

symptoms are hot flushes or sweats, which may disrupt a woman's life—wake her up three or four times a night, soaked, having to change sheets and night clothes. Other associated symptoms include depression, nervousness, irritability, a feeling as if the skin is crawling.

Q. What can estrogen do?

A. The only scientifically proven fact about estrogen replacement during menopause is that it stops flushes and sweats. There's no proof it affects the associated symptoms. In fact, we believe most other symptoms are the result of a "cascade effect." Flushes bring on insomnia, which causes fatigue, which induces nervousness. Depression is not related to hormones, in our opinion; it occurs because the menopause confronts a woman with the fact of aging.

Q. How much estrogen, then, do you give to such a woman?

A. We start her with a 1.25 milligram pill to take for the first 25 days of each month. As soon as she's stopped having flushes for two weeks, we drop the dosage, usually to .625 milligrams. On these dosages, it is necessary to add a progestational agent during the last week or ten days of treatment. After a month or two of this therapy, we reduce the estrogen to .3 milligrams and in most cases drop the progestin. We usually keep her on this prescription only during the adjustment period, about six months to a year, though some patients require long-term therapy.

Q. What are the delayed symptoms of menopause you referred to?

A. The lining of the vagina often becomes dry and fragile following menopause; this causes a burning, painful sensation during intercourse. Estrogens can correct this and associated urinary-tract problems.

Q. Are there other conditions where estrogen is helpful?

A. About five million people suffer from osteoporosis, or loss of calcium from the bones; more than three million are postmenopausal women. Hip fractures are their most common danger. Estrogens can stop the loss of calcium, at least temporarily, but they apparently can't reverse osteoporosis.

When we prescribe estrogen for this condition, we insist that our patients stop smoking, since smoking causes lung changes that interfere with calcium metabolism. We also insist that they drink three large glasses of milk a day—whole milk or skim— or take calcium gluconate tablets. And we suggest they join an exercise class, or use the Canadian Air Force exercises. Estrogens are usually given only temporarily. But the milk or calcium tablets, the exercise, and the no smoking remain lifetime needs.

Q. Do some women ask for estrogens in order to stay "feminine forever"?

A. Some do, as a result of a mistaken notion promoted by a number of doctors years ago. However, estrogens are not the fountain of youth; they won't keep the skin taut or the body firm. Besides, a post-menopausal woman is not absolutely estrogen-deficient; she merely produces less of the hormone than during her reproductive years. When her ovaries cease producing eggs, they secrete a hormone (androstenedione) which is converted to an estrogen. If the ovaries are removed, her adrenal glands produce this hormone. She doesn't need extra estrogen unless she has severe symptoms or physical signs that warrant it.

Q. Haven't current studies indicated a higher risk of endometrial cancer in women who use estrogens?

A. Yes, there is evidence that estrogen in high dosages over a long period may be associated with endometrial cancer. However, in our experience, when the smallest possible dosage is given over the shortest possible duration, no cancer has occurred. On .3 milligrams of estrogen daily—even with prolonged usage—we have yet to see evidence of any growth effect that might be a precursor of cancer. And we've been adhering to this schedule, and keeping careful records on these patients, for nearly 40 years.

So much for articles. Here also are personal letters from outstanding authorities.

From Dr. Robert N. Butler, Director, National Institute on

Aging, Bethesda, Maryland: "The treatment of the menopausal syndrome, if not effectively handled by minimal mild tranquillizing agents, may be treated by modest doses of female hormone for short periods of time."

From Dr. Robert N. Rutherford, former chief Ob/Gyn, Virginia Mason Hospital, Seattle, Washington: "The relationship of endometrial cancer to estrogen has yet to be proved. It sounds very much as if we are simply moving to a time when ladies no longer die at age forty-three as was the norm in nineteen hundred, but exist until age eighty, with resultant increase in endometrial cancer—this because of increasing age rather than any hormone influences. After twenty-five years of experience, in the low doses I give combined with a twice-a-year checkup, I believe the benefits of estrogens far outweigh the theoretical danger."

From Dr. Earle Milliard Marsh, former chief Ob/Gyn, Hazard Applachian Regional Hospital, Hazard, Kentucky: "I think that estrogen is *very safe*. If the woman has carcinoma of the breast, of course it should not be prescribed. There is some evidence, too, that if estrogen is given continuously after the menopause there may be a slight increase in the development of endometrial carcinoma. As a result, these days, we give the patient progesterone about twice a year to cause her to have an artificial period which sheds the entire endometrium. This process obviates the development of carcinoma."

From Dr. William Bickers: "You posed the question, 'Is there a relation between the replacement estrogen and cancer?' I think you have made the whole point in your question. The important word is 'replacement.' An excess of anything over and above the metabolic needs of the body, whether it be food or alcohol or estrogens, is harmful. If estrogen has any carcinogenic property at all, and I still do not think it does, it is limited to those cases in which it is abused. By abused I mean given in doses over and above the physiological requirements. This is best determined by periodic vaginal smears. As you know, I have given estrogens to my post-menopausal patients ever since 1938, but always to those in which there was a clinical and demonstrable need for replacement. Our records show that about twelve thousand women in post menopause in this office have received estrogens for at least one year or longer. Now we are beginning to see these people for follow-up examinations as they approach their later years, and our incidence of endometrial carcinoma is approximately the same in the estrogen-treated and the non-estrogen treated groups.

"I think you should particularly know that Drs. Edmund Novak and Donald Woodruff, whose book *Gynecologic and Obstetric Pathology,* is the outstanding authority in the world, have in their latest edition backed off from their earlier position condemning estrogen, and now advise its careful use. The perennial scaremonger FDA has gone, of course, to the limits of absurdity in what is and what is not carcinogenic. Nobody ever mentions the most important carcinogen—*time.* Aging was, is, and always will be the most common cause of cancer."

SUMMING UP SO FAR

So, to sum up the estrogen-cancer debate so far: The FDA has to be cautious. That is its job. You too should be cautious, since it is your body and your life. Take hormones only the way your doctor prescribes them, if he prescribes them. But remember that while it is right and good to be cautious, it is not right and good to be unduly scared.

A New Treatment

Having said all this, hold your breath! Because I recently have had word from Dr. Bickers of a new and different treatment for menopausal troubles, which was approved by the FDA in February 1980, after long success in Europe and three years of testing in the United States on over seventeen hundred women.

The new treatment is a drug called Estrovis (pronounced es-*trov*-is) and it has been approved for two reasons: it is at least as effective as conjugated estrogen, and it has little or no effect on the endometrium.

Estrovis is another form of estrogenic hormone. Remember

that all hormones are complex, or made up of different substances or fractions, just as vitamins are. There are, for instance, vitamin B_1 and vitamin B_{12}, each a fraction of vitamin B.

Estrovis is thus made from another fraction of estrogen, but it is estrogen made, not by the ovaries primarily, but by the fat and skin cells of the body. It is first stored in the body fat as a pure chemical, then gradually released from its storage place and slowly converted into estrogen. In this way, it has what doctors call a smooth therapeutic effect.

Also, since it is released and converted slowly, it does not accumulate in the blood as some hormones do; all of it that is not used is promptly thrown off. As a result, there is no need for periodic doses of progesterone to clear out the lining of the womb.

In addition, Estrovis comes in one low dose that is inexpensive and easy to remember to take. One small, pale blue tablet is taken every day for the first week; then skipped the second week, and after that only once a week on Mondays. This once-a-week dose costs about twenty-five to thirty-five cents.

"Estrovis will change the face of estrogenic therapy in America as it already has in Europe," says Dr. Bickers.

So talk over this new treatment with your doctor. Ask him to read the professional literature, and maybe let you try it.

In any event, with several modes of treatment available, you have little reason to be scared of estrogen if it is prescribed.

Go Easy on Hysterectomy

Red-haired Vera left her gynecologist's office deeply troubled. He had told her she needed a hysterectomy and, being a busy man, had said no more than that.

Just what does a hysterectomy mean? she asked herself, so upset she almost forgot to hail her bus as it came by. She'd heard it meant taking out the uterus only; then again she'd heard it meant taking out the ovaries too—even healthy ovaries sometimes. Then what were those things called "fibroids" he had mentioned? And if he did take out her ovaries, did that mean she'd have a harder or easier menopause when her time came?

She remembered as she rode along she'd been talking to a high-school principal the other night. He mentioned his wife was in the hospital having a hysterectomy, and he was sure, since they were taking out her ovaries, she would skip the menopause altogether. Avoid the whole experience, just like that. But Vera wasn't convinced.

And if this wasn't enough to confuse her, she'd been hearing a lot of talk lately saying that many hysterectomies weren't really necessary. They were just a medical racket foisted on gullible "girls." On the other hand, there were the stories that seemed to insist, "take everything the least bit suspicious out." She almost ran from the bus to her home. "Larry," she cried to her husband as she put her key in the door. "Larry, are you there? I need to talk to you right away."

Straightening Out the Terms

"Just what is a hysterectomy?" Vera wanted to know. She was confused because the word is often loosely used.

Well, it's one of several things. To be exact, it means an operation in which only the uterus or womb is taken out. The name originated a long time ago, when an ancient Greek thought that hysteria in women was somehow connected with a "wandering womb," so when you took out the womb you stopped its wandering and took out hysteria as well. So when doctors had to invent a word for its removal they hit upon the Greek word *hystera* meaning "womb," and combined it with *ectome* meaning "a cutting," and came up with hysterectomy, just as they came up with tonsillectomy for removing the tonsils. Though the old Greek theory was proved wrong a couple of centuries ago (men without wombs can be as hysterical as women) the word hysterectomy stuck.

But for removal of the ovaries there is a different term. This is oöphorectomy, and when doctors talk of removal of the uterus plus removal of the ovaries, they combine the two words and come up with hystero-oöphorectomy. When they remove the Fallopian tubes, the word they use is salpingectomy. And when tubes, ovaries, and uterus are removed, they nicely combine them all and get hystero-salpingo-oöphorectomy. And when they take out the cervix as well, they come up with pan-hystero-salpingo-oöphorectomy, *pan* meaning "all," as in Pan American.

But that kind of a thing becomes a toughie. So women as a rule lump them together into hysterectomy, using the same word no matter what is done.

I will not lump them together. Since for most of us the important distinction is between taking out the uterus only, or the uterus plus ovaries, I'll distinguish mainly between these two. I'll use the plain word "hysterectomy" for taking out the uterus only, and "complete hysterectomy" or "pan-hysterectomy" for the uterus plus ovaries, because as far as you're concerned this is what makes all the difference in the world.

The essence of the difference is this: a plain hysterectomy does not bring on a menopause. A complete or pan-hysterectomy does.

Taking out only the uterus stops menstruation permanently, as well as the ability to have children. Without a uterus to shed its lining each month, a woman can't menstruate. Without a uterus in which to grow, a baby can't develop.

But stopping menstruation and childbearing is not the crux of the matter. Some women all their lives menstruate only two or three times a year. A few occasionally skip an entire year, and I have a neighbor who skipped four years. But occasional skipping doesn't mean they have reached the menopause, since the uterus is not a key member of the gland network and it is the glandular changes that bring the menopause about. But the ovaries *are* a key number. When they are removed a glandular readjustment does take place, and the changing years suddenly arrive. Now this sudden loss is often extremely upsetting if you're as young as twenty or thirty. That's because when you're that young, your body and emotions are nowhere near set for losing your ovarian hormones. So both emotionally and physically, young women sometimes have a rather rough time adjusting to a surgical change.

But it's much less upsetting if you're in your late forties, because then you are set. You can, in a sense, compare a pan-hysterectomy at an early age with bearing a seven-month baby, and compare a pan-hysterectomy at a later age with bearing a full-term baby. In one instance nature isn't ready for the event, and complications almost always arise. In the other, nature is ready; complications may or may not occur.

Past fifty, we used to think a surgical change was apt not to be upsetting at all because by then you are quite certain to be ready for ovarian loss. But surgeons who observe carefully have discovered this isn't always true.

Dr. William Bickers tells me that not long ago he removed ovaries from two women aged sixty and sixty-five. Neither of them had menstruated in fifteen years or had a single flush. Surprisingly enough at their age, both were thrown into violent flushes and other menopausal symptoms as soon as their still-functioning ovaries were taken out.

So instead of making you skip the changing years, removing both ovaries does the opposite. It brings them on with a bang.

WHY DO THEY DO IT?

Yet here's a paradox: Many doctors remove ovaries from women over forty-five as a matter of course while doing a hysterectomy.

Why? Not every doctor is callous and does a pan-hysterectomy as a "racket" in the sense of looking for a larger fee. Once he's operating anyway, almost no surgeon charges more for a complete hysterectomy than for a plain one, even though it's a much more complex operation to do.

Nor does he do it to be "mean." He does it because it is according to his best judgment. And if he has sincerely altered that judgment while you were under anesthesia on the operating table, he couldn't exactly wake you up, ring for tea, and chat with you while asking your permission to do more. Moreover, once you have signed permission for any operation, it means that, ethically and legally, you have put yourself in his experienced hands and are trusting him to do the best job he can.

No, many surgeons who have taken out ovaries during a hysterectomy have done so for special reasons.

First, they observed that while women in their forties often suffered more in a menopause brought on by surgery, this wasn't always the case. They got a jolt, to be sure, but they weren't always aware of it. Like with a slower and more normal change, some women walked calmly through the experience, tossing it little more than a passing thought. And again, as with a normal change, in a fairly short time a readjustment took place. The seesaw became balanced, things equaled out, and they felt pretty much their cheerful selves again. Therefore, since most hysterectomies are done after forty, a noticeable upset wasn't always in the cards.

Moreover, they knew that these days when a noticeable upset did occur the powerful proven help of man-made hormones was available. In a surgical change over forty, a few more of these might be needed or for a little longer. In the twenties or thirties, much more and for much longer. But they were ready and to hand.

But what motivated them most was that they really believed the ovaries were useless in a woman once the childbearing years were past. In fact, they were worse than useless, they might stir up later trouble. Why keep in something that could stir up mischief, yet was headed for the shelf?

The possible later trouble they feared most was ovarian cancer. Many doctors seriously figured the possibility of ovarian cancer developing years later was justification for removing healthy ovaries while they had the chance. Cancer is a dread disease. During an operation on any genital organ, they were "in the neighborhood," so to speak. Why make a woman maybe come running back when they could make a clean sweep?

Another, more common, trouble they feared was the development of ovarian cysts. Cysts are little sacs of fluid, and they sometimes develop later because even simple hysterectomy can deprive the ovaries of about one third of their blood supply, and with the blood supply cut, cysts can result. Or sometimes tiny ovarian cysts that can't be seen by the most careful examination are present at the time of the operation. In a few years these too may grow and require a second operation—an operation that is usually more difficult than the first.

TIMES HAVE CHANGED

Yes, those were the reasons doctors once used for removing ovaries, and pretty sturdy reasons they seemed.

Then around 1947 things began to change. New positive evidence for keeping them in began to leap to light.

Distinguished surgeons like Dr. Henry Falk, former chief of obstetrics and gynecology at the French Hospital in New York, stated: "I no longer take out healthy ovaries unless the woman specifically requests it. I haven't done so for the past ten years." And all over the country other doctors began declaring the same.

They were saying this because man-made hormones, while valuable, were found to be not quite as valuable as one's own. But most of all because the "useless" ovaries were beginning to give evidence of being not nearly as useless as had been thought.

And as to being useless, Dr. Clyde Randall, professor of gynecology at the University of Buffalo Medical School, was one of the first to have a hunch this might prove to be an exaggeration. He got his hunch from the fact, long puzzling to many people, that women these days live much longer than men. What, he asked, could be the cause of this longer life? In most bodily blessings, men and women are roughly equal. The main difference lies in their hormones. Women have more estrogen than men. And this estrogen is made mainly by our ovaries. Could some ovarian hormone be made right on into old age and have something to do with our tendency to a longer life? It was a fascinating thought.

What Dr. Randall did was this: Knowing that one way of detecting the presence of natural estrogen is by examination of the vaginal cells, he and his associates at the school took samples of such cells from 1,473 women in or long past their period of changing years. Some were in their forties, some as old as sixty-five. All had stopped menstruating at least a year before, and as an added precaution none had received estrogen in the form of medicine for at least six months.

He carefully examined the cells of these women. His hunch was right! More than half of the women did show evidence of natural estrogen still being made within their own bodies, some for as long as fifteen years after menstruation had totally ceased.

In an exciting paper read before the Eightieth Annual Meeting of the American Gynecological Society in September 1957, Dr. Randall reported:

> One to two years after they had spontaneously stopped menstruating, 171 women were still making the natural female hormone.
>
> Two to five years later, 108 women were still producing estrogen.

One hundred and twenty-one women were at it more than fifteen years later.

It added up to a grand total of 812 women of all those studied, or fifty-five percent, continuing to produce ovarian hormone for years after their menopause had arrived. True, the amount of estrogen in some was slight. But in some it was moderate and in some marked. And it totaled that unexpected, surprising fifty-five percent.

This still didn't prove the estrogen was coming from their ovaries, however, for estrogen, like androgen, is also made by our adrenal glands.

His next job, therefore, was to separate the women who had their ovaries from those who didn't. Now he compared the slides of 112 women who'd had a complete hysterectomy with those of 183 women who'd had a plain hysterectomy. About thirty percent more women whose ovaries had been preserved when the uterus was removed showed a persistence of estrogen effect. This estrogen had to be coming partly from the left-in ovaries. Those "useless" ovaries indeed!

WHY IT'S IMPORTANT

But what's important about a persistence of estrogen? Why care? These were the next pressing questions. Dr. Randall answered them too.

Estrogen, as we know, is not only a sex hormone; it is a generally stimulating, protective hormone. In older women it appears to do important protective jobs. It helps to protect from arteriosclerosis or hardening of the arteries. It helps to protect from osteoporosis, or loss of calcium from the bones. It preserves the softness and elasticity of the vaginal tissues essential to the normal enjoyment of sex.

Hypertension, for instance, is found in only thirteen percent of women who show a moderate to marked persistence of estrogen. Those without it show much more. Arteriosclerosis, according to some studies, is from ten percent to forty-five percent higher in women who have lost their ovaries than in those who have not.

And since estrogen is a skin-nourisher, a rather odd effect of ovarian removal can be a sudden allergic skin reaction. Maybe because of the sudden change in body chemistry, maybe just because the stress of the operation in general, but women who have never been allergic before can become allergic now.

Take the case of Madge. Right in the hospital immediately after a complete hysterectomy Madge became allergic to the rubber on the back of adhesive tape. Since adhesive tape is used most liberally to support one's "middle" at such a time, she broke out in blisters all over her abdomen and back. But it didn't stop there. The allergy traveled through her blood stream, and came out in unexpected places on her body. She soon became allergic to the rubber in her girdle and brassiere. Any place rubber touched her became red and inflamed; even rubber from so seemingly innocent thing as a Band-Aid. Especially in hot weather, a Band-Aid left its clear outline on her skin . . . and did it itch!

But the allergy lasted for only about a year. Then as her body readjusted and got used to its new chemistry, it took its leave as suddenly as it had come. She could use adhesive tape again and go back to her old brassieres and girdle, which luckily she hadn't thrown out.

Then there was Helen, who developed a different allergy. Helen had been dyeing her hair for as long as she could remember. She dyed it as usual after a pan-hysterectomy. Lo! She, too, broke out all over her face and scalp. She didn't wait for readjustment; she let her hair go permanently gray, which proved most becoming. The rash cleared up.

Dr. Falk and Dr. Randall concur in the importance of the ovaries in post-menopausal women. Dr. Falk says: "The ovaries after the age of forty-five still give off some form of internal secretion which is essential. Their removal causes changes—among them emotional ones—that are difficult to explain."

Today many informed surgeons take the age of forty-five as a dividing line and arrange women on either side of that line this way:

Under the age of forty-five, they remove ovaries during hysterectomy only if they are definitely diseased.

Around or over the age of forty-five, they remove them if they believe that the ovaries are likely to become diseased.

By "become diseased" they mean likely to develop cancer.

The Northampton surgeon Dr. Samuel Topal says: "Cancer of the ovary happens to only one percent of all women, but it's a dreadful cancer when it does. It rarely gives an early warning. Because of its location, the ovary is hard to feel, and its symptoms, like those of digestive upsets, are very vague." So if a woman is around age forty-five, Dr. Topal figures that her ovaries have only a functioning life left of five or six years. To play safe therefore he usually takes them out. And if she is already fifty, he almost surely takes them out and immediately puts her on a low dose of estrogen. It is not always necessary to continue the estrogen however, because women's bodies are so complex and miraculous that, as mentioned in the last chapter, in many cases their fat and skin cells begin to secrete a substance that is converted to estrogen. Indeed, in very fat women so much may be secreted by their cells they become a more serious candidate for cancer than they otherwise would be. Another argument for keeping one's figure reasonably slim.

On the other hand, Dr. William Bickers does not believe that ovaries that might become cancerous should come out. He believes in leaving in both ovaries, one ovary, or at least a piece of an ovary. Even a piece of an ovary is important since it may continue to produce enough estrogen to make it possible to sail through the menopause without any trouble at all.

So here you are: Some doctors, like Dr. Topal, think that if a woman around forty-five is having a hysterectomy, her ovaries should come out along with her uterus. Other doctors, like Dr. Bickers, believe they should be left in.

TALK IT OVER WITH YOUR DOCTOR

If you are around forty-five and your gynecologist has suggested a hysterectomy and you're not sure what should be done, be fair to him and yourself. Talk the matter over with him.

And if you find out he does believe in taking out your ovaries, tell him politely that you'd like to discuss the matter with someone else as well. And make that doctor the finest you can find. If you don't know how to find a top specialist, call up the hospital in your neighborhood with the best reputation and ask for the names of the doctors on their gynecology staff. Or if there happens to be a medical school nearby, call there and ask the dean for the names of the best professors in the subject.

If neither of these is possible, ask your original gynecologist to recommend someone. He may be glad to tell you, provided you are willing to see someone at least equal to himself. A doctor welcomes another opinion if he feels it's as good as his own—in fact, it often secretly relieves him of responsibility he was reluctant to take by himself.

Certainly all this double-checking may take time and money. But can you think of a better way of being reasonably sure of what should be done to your own insides?

SPEAK UP

But it's more than time or money that stops some of us. It's because we're just plain frightened. Frightened of questioning a doctor—especially a surgeon with a princely air! For he represents "father" to us, and out of old childish habit we daren't speak up. Also, once we've started with one doctor we sort of feel he owns us, anyway for the problem in hand.

Dr. Walter C. Alvarez, emeritus consultant in medicine at the Mayo Clinic, reminds us such feelings are foolish. A doctor, he says, doesn't own the patient any more than the patient owns the doctor. Certainly it's good to feel he's a father whom you can trust. But it's also good to feel yourself a grownup who can talk back calmly when you must.

So if any doctor scares the daylights out of you, gather your wits together. Speak up! Arrive at his office with a written list of questions. Then grab him by the mental coattails and insist he answer them. If the questions are intelligent, far from offending him, he may develop for you a sneaking respect.

A friend of mine, a teacher named Sylvia, learned to speak up the hard way.

All during the nine months of her first pregnancy Sylvia was too terrified of her obstetrician to ask him if he believed in anesthesia during childbirth. She didn't find out until she was in labor that he did not. He was a "nature boy" to the extreme. Beg as she might, she couldn't get more than an aspirin and a pep talk, though she had one of those excruciating labors that go on and on.

Next time she was smarter. She didn't even let herself *get* pregnant until she had talked herself out with a new doctor and found he figured things the other way round.

Maybe one of the best ideas is to take along a friend when you go to see a doctor, because even if he's not the frightening kind, the very visit touches off feelings of vulnerability and weakness since for so long women have been brushed off with a "there, there, little woman. Just leave everything to me."

The best kind of friend to take is a health-care professional. Sometimes even she may not be able to speak up completely; nurses aren't as a rule trained that way. But she'll at least give you moral support.

Plain Hysterectomy

Now to plain hysterectomy, or taking out the uterus alone.

Most hysterectomies are done for fibroids of the uterus. But fibroids aren't as dangerous as we may have heard. Small fibroids are so common in the forties as to be almost normal. About a third of all women have them before menopause time.

Fibroids are lumps of excess tissue. They are usually called benign, meaning harmless, tumors. When they stay small and do not cause symptoms, they do not endanger either health or life.

No one knows the cause of fibroids or why they sometimes do, and more often do not, cause symptoms. No one knows either why they tend to start in the twenties and thirties and reach their peak in the forties.

But the fact that they can happen to many women is such good news it's worth memorizing. *Small fibroids that do not cause symptoms are so common around the time of the menopause as to be practically normal. If they stay small and continue not to give symptoms, they are no indication for a hasty hysterectomy.*

Meet two gentlemen: Dr. Robert T. Frank, former chief of obstetrics and gynecology at Mt. Sinai Hospital in New York, and Dr. Alan F. Guttmacher, former president of Planned Parenthood.

Dr. Frank is speaking: "After fifty years of practice, I took 916 fibroid cases at random and made a special study of them. Most had been referred to me by other doctors as needing immediate surgery. But I decided to watch and wait. It turned out half of them didn't need the operation at all, especially if they were around the menopausal age. And of this half, only five women needed it right away."

Dr. Guttmacher is speaking: "Fibroids are not dangerous and do not have to be removed in most cases. And when they do, there is seldom need for haste."

Here's more good news: Small fibroids that develop in the late thirties or forties not only tend to stay small, they tend to shrink and disappear once the changing years have set in. They do this disappearing act à la Houdini, because during the menopause you lose much of the natural estrogen that was stimulating them to grow. Also, as your estrogen goes down, your androgen or male hormone goes comparatively up, and this tends to shrink them further. For the same reason, new fibroids seldom come along.

Dr. Lawrence R. Wharton, emeritus professor of gynecology at Johns Hopkins Medical School in Baltimore, makes the statement: "I have seen fibroid tumors as large as cantaloupes become as small as marbles during the menopause. In some such cases the patients had refused hysterectomy which I myself advised, and I have had the privilege of following them and seeing the tumors practically disappear."

SOME HAVE TO COME OUT

Of course not all of them disappear. Some fibroids do start acting up and have to come out eventually. But these are basically limited to three instances.

Dr. Guttmacher lists these three.

1. Fibroids should come out when, instead of staying small, they start to grow and become larger than a uterus containing an unborn baby three months old.

2. Fibroids should come out when they cause pressure symptoms; that is, press hard on bladder, rectum, or abdomen.

3. Fibroids should come out when they make you bleed so heavily and so often that you become anemic by actual test, and this anemia is severe enough to present a danger to health.

Now you can't very well judge for yourself the size of your uterus. But you can judge when a fibroid is beginning to press on your abdomen, because then you will feel a large, hard, protruding mass no girdle will pull in. You can also judge pressure on your bladder or rectum because then you'll have constantly and unbearably to "go."

As for abnormal bleeding, you can judge this too by keeping a diary. This means carefully recording your menstrual periods and noting if they get heavier and heavier each month without light periods between. Heavy periods that alternate with light periods are part of the normal menopausal pattern. These will not make you anemic as a rule. Vitamins with a small iron supplement—the cheapest you can buy—should take care of them. It's most cheering to remember that the loss of blood in an average menstrual period is only around three tablespoonfuls. Unless the flow becomes regularly much heavier, and keeps on coming much more frequently than usual, it's not something you need to do something about in haste.

REGULAR CHECKUPS NEEDED

Obviously, don't neglect your regular checkups. Don't neglect watching for the possible development of cancer of the uterus, either.

The sane way to do this, according to Dr. Wharton, is to take a twice-a-year Pap test. This is a recognized cancer-detection test in which a few drops of vaginal secretion are taken and examined under a microscope to see if they test normal or abnormal. Even if they do test abnormal, that doesn't mean you should ring a fire alarm, because not all abnormal reports mean there are serious problems. Sometimes a mere inflammation or infection—which will clear up—will yield test results that are abnormal. Only if the report suggests definite cell changes toward cancer, changes your doctor will recognize, do you need to follow up with these further tests: A biopsy, in which a tiny piece of tissue from the lining of the uterus is taken out and examined, and which can usually be done right in the doctor's office. Or a dilatation and curettage, familiarly called a D and C, in which a sample of the entire uterus lining is gently scraped out and examined, though this is usually done in a hospital. Or, often best of all, an examination under anesthesia, which is not the same as an operation but which brings about such a dramatic relaxation of the genital organs that your doctor gets an almost breathtakingly different feel of them than he gets in an ordinary exam.

THE VILLAIN IS HASTE

By now you must have guessed what causes most of the unnecessary hysterectomies, about which you may have become alarmed. It is haste. And haste and a racket are two different things.

Most doctors are conscientious; years of training have made them so. More, they are the only profession outside the priesthood bound by a solemn oath to do no harm.

They are also constantly journeying to medical meetings to

exchange information and improve themselves. (There was recently a three-day conference in New York on the uterus alone.) And there are such heaps of medical journals that a doctor could hole up in a corner and do nothing but read them all day long.

But doctors are also part of the times we live in. And the sore finger of our age is speed. We don't walk across streets, we leap across them, even though when we get across all we do is stare vacantly into a shop window. We don't drive cars leisurely, we race them, even on a Sunday ride-to-nowhere. And in a restaurant, if a waiter doesn't trip over his feet and rush to serve us before we've even decided what to eat, we drum the table like maniacs.

So when we get panicky over an innocent fibroid tumor, doctors can get panicky also. Instead of "When in doubt, don't," their motto can become "When in doubt, do." And with total honesty and no thought of fee on the doctor's part, our uteruses and ovaries can be sacrificed as a result.

Then there's an additional and subtle force pulling at surgeons, in particular. Everybody enjoys doing what he does well, especially when there's an audience to applaud him. Doesn't a good actor like to act even without pay? Doesn't a good cook like to cook even though she gives the cake away? Surgeons these days perform very well indeed. And there are a large number of assistants in a modern operating room who, no matter how many masks they are wearing or how busy they are, have time to applaud the chief with their eyes.

But what probably influences surgeons most is the fact that many are really convinced the uterus is useless once the childbearing days are past. The ovaries may still have some kind of job. The uterus is a once-faithful race horse ready to retire to grass.

If all this weren't enough, there's a type of woman who almost pushes a surgeon. She has a few small fibroids plus a great many vague complaints, complaints as vague as "dizziness," and some doctor in desperation has told her a hysterectomy might cure her. Or, she's just plain impatient with normally heavy bleedings and she'll do anything to stop them; anything! She arrives at the surgeon's office with her mind made up. She'll have her uterus out right away. When he hesitates, she practically begs for an operation, and it's a strong man who can resist. Especially when he can shrug his shoulders and say to himself, "At her age, what harm can it do?"

Well, what harm *can* it do? What's wrong with removing a soon-to-retire uterus along with a few non-pesky fibroids, or to try to cure some general vague complaints?

The answer is, emotional harm. Psychological harm. No modern woman can overlook these.

Many years ago two doctors in Chicago, Dr. William S. Kroger and Dr. I. S. Freed, wrote a thought-provoking book called *Psychosomatic Gynecology*. Drs. Kroger and Freed insist that all operations carry a great emotional shock, but one involving the lower abdomen carries about the most. That's because our genital organs are in the lower abdomen. And our genital organs are a central part of the picture we carry around of ourselves as complete human beings.

Surgeons have long known men carry such a picture. None of them would dream of tampering with a man's genital organs, even if he were eighty years old, without realizing he would be shaken to the depths. They sometimes forget a woman can be almost as shaken too.

You can lose, say, your gall bladder from your upper abdomen with little regret. But your gall bladder wasn't you. Unless it was very obstreperous, in daily life you hardly gave it a thought. But for about thirty years you've had to think of your genital organs at least once a month during menstruation, and much more during the nine months of pregnancy. So, like a cherished wedding dress wrapped away in tissue paper, your ovaries and uterus have come to symbolize femininity. Even when their services seem over, you can't lose them without a deep wrench.

DIFFERENT IN A NORMAL MENOPAUSE

All this is quite different in a normal menopause. Then they fade out slowly, gradually, over a period of months or years. You have time to get used to a new picture of yourself, as you've gradually been getting used to other new pictures all your life. But with surgery it's a matter of minutes. You go under the anesthetic one way and wake up another. They're whisked away so fast, it's as my grandmother used to jokingly put it, "Now you see me; now you ain't."

Eventually, even after surgery, you get used to their absence. You repaint the picture as quickly as nature readjusts your body. It's just harder to do, that's all.

I know that I myself broke down and wept when I had a pan-hysterectomy. I cried, "They were *my* ovaries and I loved them!" In a few weeks I got over my anguish, just as women get over post-partum depression. In a few months new hormones began to replace the old. I even came to be grateful to my doctor for doing what he was convinced was right. Still, I didn't cry when I lost my appendix. Was it because I didn't think of my appendix as such a central part of *me*?

USE YOUR WITS

So use every sane bit of sense you have before consenting to, or begging for, a hysterectomy. Consult two gynecological specialists. (Blue Cross now tries to insist on this before they pay out, because they have found that when there are two opinions the number of operations drops sharply.) Accept without panic the presence of small fibroids that are not causing symptoms. If still in doubt, ask for a dilatation and curettage, biopsy, or an examination under anesthesia which is much more thorough than the ordinary kind.

And if after all this the decision is still that an operation is in order, ask your surgeon what he thinks is the *most* he may do. Then start drawing a new portrait of yourself immediately. If he does a lot, it won't be so much of a shock. If he does less, you'll be happily surprised.

LITTLE CHANGE IN SEX LIFE

Draw the portrait, too, so it includes yourself as a woman able to receive about the same pleasure in sex as before. Here again, though, a distinction must be made between a plain hysterectomy and a complete.

In a plain hysterectomy, when only the uterus goes, little pleasure goes. In a complete hysterectomy, when the ovaries go too, more pleasure goes because the vagina becomes drier and lubricating jelly is usually needed. Susanne Morgan, a woman who had a necessary complete hysterectomy at the age of twenty-nine and told her story in a pamphlet written in collaboration with the Boston Women's Health Collective, said she felt less pleasure because she felt the loss of uterine contractions in connection with her orgasms, and also found her orgasms less intense. Said Ms. Morgan: "I've noticed sexual changes and I feel bitter, even though I know I'm in charge of my sexuality, and it is certainly better than when my uterus *hurt* with orgasms . . . I also miss the sudden feelings of wetness that took me by surprise . . . My husband and I are having trouble relearning how to get me aroused. I feel cheated, since sex was so good for me before, and I need to remind myself how powerful and sexy I really am."

Bitterness is not her sole reaction, however. "Since the hysterectomy I am much happier and in a better place in my life. But I still feel anger and grief and fear. My work in re-evaluation co-counseling has been very helpful in giving me space to feel those feelings, yet not let them rule my life."

Maybe that's the answer—you too will probably feel ambivalent for a while. You will feel a mixture of anger, fear, grief, and happiness. Happiness because possibly you have strong religious feelings about not using contraceptives, and after a hysterectomy you no longer need to use them. Grief because you cannot have any more children. Fear that gives you twinges of feeling that in some way you are no longer like other women, or that your husband will in some way be put off.

ANOTHER WOMAN'S STORY

Another woman, we shall call Mary Foley, also felt ambivalent after a hysterectomy, mainly because she did not know what to expect.

I report it as she wrote it: "I asked for a complete hysterectomy because I had fibroids that were growing and pressing on my other organs, as well as ovaries that were giving me pain. Also I was fifty-three years old. Still, I did not expect the operation to be so emotionally and psychologically devastating. It is devastating because no time is spent in advance preparing the patient for the effects of the surgery. The operation is painful after the fact, since there is physical pain from the incision and pain from the gas which ensues. This makes the first few days uncomfortable, to put it mildly.

"Then sudden removal of estrogen can create hot flashes, and give you headaches which are severe enough to demand medication and cause loss of sleep. Also there is depression, and this causes crying and the general feeling of being sorry for yourself. Finally there is much debate over whether to give supplemental estrogen and it looks like you are damned if you do, and damned if you don't.

"But wait a minute, who tells you all this? You find out by reading everything you can get your hands on when you get home —after the fact.

"If you complain about the flashes, the headache, the crying jags, you get a prescription for estrogen with instructions to take as little as possible to control the symptoms. If you complain about constipation, burning urination, or trouble in these areas, you are told 'we moved a few things around down there,' or merely 'you did have major surgery, what can you expect?'

"I am of the opinion that if there were more women gynecologists there would be more compassionate answers.

"My own son is studying to be a doctor, and should he specialize in gyn/ob, I shall give him the wherewithall to understand all this.

"When I am asked about the operation I say 'it is like being hit with a Mack truck and recovering from it.'"

But Mary is a strong-spirited and positive-thinking person, and she made the best of a difficult time. When I saw her shortly after her operation, she was smiling and cheerful and looked marvelous. She was back teaching physical education, and was proud that her doctor had let her go back to work in five weeks instead of the usual six because she was so wonderfully fit.

MEN VERSUS WOMEN DOCTORS

One point Mary made is worthy of more discussion. This is the matter of going to a woman gynecologist instead of a man. Even finding a woman surgeon if possible.

A few years ago finding a woman surgeon was very difficult; only ten percent of hospital Ob/Gyn surgical residents were women. But according to Dr. Samuel Topal, now twenty-five percent are women. And he believes the figure will be up to fifty percent soon.

When I asked him, a little doubtfully, if women had the stamina to be surgeons since surgeons must stand on their feet for many long hours, he answered: "Certainly they have the stamina. In many ways they really are the stronger sex."

The answer is to find a doctor with whom you are comfortable. I have had male doctors who were compassionate and caring, and others who were arrogant. One arrogant surgeon explained his coldness by saying "Sympathy you get from your friends, authority you get only from me."

I have also had kind women doctors and unsympathetic, bad-tempered women doctors. It is one of those personal matters you must decide for yourself.

REACTIONS OF MEN

Back to Susanne Morgan who was also greatly concerned about men's reaction to hysterectomy. Writes Ms. Morgan: "How do men react to hysterectomy? Very little is written, but what is mentioned is that some men have very strong reactions. Several studies discuss women whose mates leave them after hysterectomy, taunt them with being 'half a woman,' or 'neutered,' or refuse to have intercourse with them. These are the exceptions, and most men treat their wives tenderly after hysterectomy."

My husband was one who was tender. When I became allergic to the rubber on the back of adhesive tape after my hysterectomy, he ran all over town to find me a special soothing oil the doctor recommended, and bound my arms lightly at night with gauze so I wouldn't scratch them while I slept.

Ms. Morgan agrees also that sex is a wonderful combination of the physical and the emotional. No matter what happens, a woman can give and receive tenderness after any operation, especially if she has built up the memory of tenderness received and shared. Indeed, the sharing can become even finer as she and her husband are drawn together in a new understanding bond.

MANY "IF'S" AND "BUT'S"

Obviously, there are many "if's" and "but's" about hysterectomy. Here are some others.

Most doctors, as I said, are conscientious. But some are not. Some are extremely money-minded. As one Ob/Gyn quoted by the New York *Times* admitted: "Since the birth rate is falling some of us aren't making the living we did previously, so out comes a uterus or two to pay the rent." (Interestingly, far fewer hysterectomies are performed for the sake of money in Great Britain, which is under the National Health Plan, than are done in America. As British surgeons are on salary, they have no pecuniary interest in operating unnecessarily. Also, such operations are scrutinized more carefully there. When in doubt, the government refuses to pay.)

In a New York *Times* review of a book called *Women's Health Care, the Hidden Malpractice,* the reviewer, Alix Nelson, tells how some doctors have been known to work on the scare principle, and try to talk a woman into a hysterectomy by telling her that "removing your uterus now will save you from the risk of developing cancer there later." Ms. Nelson says this even happened to her, and the doctor didn't tell her that the death rate from cancer of the uterus is much lower than that from hysterectomy.

Altogether, according to Dr. John Bunker of Stanford University, far too many hysterectomies are being performed in the United States these days. A full seventy-five thousand more women had them in 1977 than in 1975, and a third of these in his opinion were probably unnecessary.

They occurred because women had been talked into them for flimsy reasons, or were in teaching hospitals where medical students were learning to do hysterectomies and so needed patients, and mysteriously they were done far more in certain parts of the country than in others, though presumably the health of women is the same everywhere.

THE COURAGE TO STAND STILL

There are many times in life when we need courage, courage to go forward, as well as courage of another kind. The famous singer, Lotte Lehmann, says the most valuable lesson she ever learned was the courage to stand still. The courage to stand still can be golden in contemplating hysterectomy. To stand still while repeated medical checkups show small fibroids are not getting bigger. To wait it out while normally heavy bleedings seem unbearable, until one day your body in its wisdom bids them be gone. The courage to speak up and ask questions galore.

Courage can be golden, too, if you've already had an operation and are tempted to think you didn't need it. Now you'll want to decide it probably *was* necessary and not look back and blame a very human surgeon for doing what he did. He may have saved you from a second and more difficult operation. He may have done even better. He may have performed a modern miracle and saved your life.

16

Looking Forward

If you are about forty when you read this, you have almost twice as much time in which to stay alive as an adult as you have already had.

That's a rather startling statement, isn't it? Almost twice as much time left for being an adult as before! Well, figure it out.

From age zero to age twenty you were a child, a schoolgirl, an adolescent—a cocoon that had not opened up. Then came the great birthday of twenty. You became an adult; for the first time entered the grown-up world. For the next twenty years you stayed in that world, working, hoping, breathing its fine air—a woman now. Then you became forty. What can you look forward to? You can look forward to staying alive to about seventy-seven. And from forty to seventy-seven gives you over thirty-five years in which to continue in the adult world, or almost twice as long as you have already had.

What is more, you are the first woman in history to be this lucky. Things were quite different not so long ago. As short a time as three hundred years ago the life expectancy of the average woman was seventeen years. Yes, that's equally startling—seventeen compared to seventy-seven. But when the Pilgrims were setting sail for the American shores, a newborn baby girl could be expected to live to be only seventeen years of age. That was the average, of course, and took in all those who died in infancy and youth. But between the lack of sanitation and ignorance of medicine in general, that was all one could expect. A few women lived on to menopausal age and beyond, but they were the exception—rare persons indeed. No wonder people didn't pay much attention to the menopause in those days. Few women lived long enough to experience it.

Then matters began to improve, though slowly. By the time of the American Civil War, or around 1860, a woman's life expectancy had more than doubled. She could now look forward to living to the age of forty, which was much better than seventeen.

By 1900 things were even better. Eight more years had been added. Instead of forty, she could now achieve forty-eight.

And then came the really remarkable spurt—the spurt of our own twentieth century. From 1900 to 1979 a full twenty-nine and a half years were added, the biggest jump in history. For the first time since the Bible was written, the idea of threescore and ten was more of a reality than a dream. In 1979 a woman could expect to live to more than seventy-seven years.

But that *still* doesn't tell the whole story.

Exciting as seventy-seven sounds, remember again it means expectancy at birth. It is always the deaths in childhood and youth that bring the average down. If you have weathered these pitfalls and are alive and kicking and fairly sound in your forties, then your expectancy is even greater than the average. For the longer you have already lived, the longer you will live, up to a point. The figures run like this:

If you are now forty-five, you can expect another thirty-two years on the average, or a life of more than seventy-seven.

If you are now fifty-five, you can expect another twenty-four years, or a life of more than seventy-nine.

If you are now sixty-five, you can expect another fifteen and a half years, or a life of eighty or more.

If you are now seventy-five, you can expect an average of another nine, or a grand total of eighty-four.

With new health aids being discovered every day—penicillin, aureomycin, streptomycin, mineral supplements—who knows what the future may bring? Certainly the odds for a long and healthy life are getting better every day. As someone has put it, "There are now more younger older people than ever before!"

OLD MYTHS

What are you going to do with this gift of long life now that you have it? I'm going to say pooh to a lot of old myths!

There is, for instance, the myth that the loss of physical power we all suffer from to some degree as we get older, means a loss of happiness as well.

This is not true. We are not necessarily unhappy because we can't jog for five miles, or take a ten-mile hike. We may enjoy a short walk or a morning of gardening just as much. We are not necessarily unhappy because we can't accept an invitation to an all-night party because we will be too tired the next day. Or drive twenty miles to a movie over an icy winter road. We are not unhappy because by now we know that it's no fun to get over-tired; and that, if we wait, we'll get invited to a party that ends at a reasonable hour. Or that the movie will probably appear in a nearby theater so we'll only have to drive three miles.

I once read an essay called "The Joys of Not Going." I remember that essay every time I say "I'll take a rain-check on the late-night party," or think up a quick excuse for not doing something else that doesn't make sense, and settle down to staying home instead.

Then there's a myth around that, as we age, we will suffer a sharp decline in our intellectual powers. That we will not be able to learn new things as easily as before, or maybe not learn them at all. I say pooh again! Alex Comfort tells of an Australian experiment with a group of seventy-year-olds who were studying German, which was for them a brand-new language. They learned as fast as a group of fifteen-year-olds, and what is more, they got the same good marks on their tests.

They did this because they had more experience in learning, as well as a better vocabulary and a better mental "filing system." Remember that wheeze "You can't teach an old dog new tricks?"

This group simply laughed it off because they knew they were people, not dogs.

BAD IMAGE

Next, I'm going to fight the bad image society has foisted on older people when it sees them as fragile, senile, sexless, or weak in the head. I'm going to come back with a firm "no" when someone tells me that senility is inevitable because I know it isn't. My grandmother never became the least bit senile. At eighty-six we brought her a black hat as a present to go strolling in. "I don't want a black hat; I want a stunnish red hat!" she exclaimed. (Yes, she said "stunnish." She also thanked the "Old Mighty" for blessings, and spoke of her "hot blood pressure.") And she died at eighty-seven quietly in her sleep.

My mother also died quietly at the age of ninety-three. She was on occasion a tiny bit senile, if you can call it senility. When I went to see her one day she said pleasantly, "Thank you for coming on my birthday." "It isn't your birthday; it's Washington's birthday," I replied. "Oh well," she answered cheerfully, "I knew it was somebody's birthday." Later, when I thought of it, I recalled her own birthday was only a few days off.

Remember that the people who do become senile pile up in nursing homes where everyone sees them and talks about them, so that their numbers become greatly exaggerated.

MAKE WAVES

More, I'm going to prove that I'm not weak in the head by continuing to "make waves." By "making waves" I mean that when there's a cause worth fighting for, I'll fight. I'll write letters to my local newspapers and to my congressmen. I'll walk in protest marches if I have to, as Alice Paul, the ninety-year-old suffragette, did for the ERA. In other words, I'll refuse to "grow old gracefully," which usually means "grow old silently," something many people would like us to do in order to keep us nothing more than cookie-bakers.

The poet Dylan Thomas probably expressed this best when he wrote: "Do not go gentle into that good night." I'll be gentle sometimes, but only sometimes. At other times I'll be assertive, and I'll be the one to decide which times I'll be which.

For assertiveness mainly boils down to not giving up. And people who don't give up have a much better chance of succeeding at anything they do.

Here are some other experiments that prove this.

A group of rats were shut into a cage from which they could escape by pushing a special button that would open the cage door, but they were not shown where that special button was. At the same time another group was shut into a cage but *were* shown the location of the button. When the second group began to feel hopelessly enclosed, they pushed the button and escaped. But the first group, not knowing the location of the button, gave up, and began to run around in a state of great fear until their keeper let them out.

To double-check, a similar experiment was done with a group of children who were locked into rooms whose doors also had escape buttons, but were not told of the existence of such buttons, while a second group was locked into rooms and shown where escape buttons could be found. The children who knew how to get out pushed the buttons and ran out; the ones who didn't know there were any gave up, sat still, and piteously cried.

Women have often been made to believe there were no escape buttons, that nothing could be done to change their lives. If they were poor, they had to remain poor. If they got pregnant every year, they had to cope with it, even if they became so ill they died as a result. Anything that locked them into such situations was something they had to accept as "God's will."

But not all women accepted. Take the photographer Imogene Cunningham.

Ms. Cunningham seemed hopelessly poor. But she knew that at least she could take pictures. She scrounged up the money in 1910, while still a high-school student, and took a corre-

spondence course in photography. By the time she graduated she
was so confident she borrowed more money and opened her own
portrait studio. Though she married a few years later and had
two children, that didn't phase her; she continued to manage to
work hard both at home and in her studio. At home she specialized in pictures of the flowers she grew in her own garden; in her
studio she did increasingly sophisticated portrait-studies of children and friends, studies that brought her enough recognition to
have several one-woman shows. At the age of eighty-six she was
still at it. She won a Guggenheim grant to study abroad, and was
still working when she died at ninety-three.

Obviously, nobody ever made Ms. Cunningham believe that
because she was a woman she couldn't have both a career and a
family, so she simply went ahead and did.

I have a feeling that, along with confidence, Ms. Cunningham was not afraid to get old. Many people are afraid, especially around the birthdays that mark the end of one decade and
the start of another. They are seized with a sudden fear that from
now on all will be downhill.

But most people who get such feelings of fear get over them
—if they have the courage to fall apart then pick themselves up
and put themselves together again.

Listen to Jane Fonda talking to a newspaper reporter in
1977: "I was terrified when I turned thirty. I was pregnant and
had the mumps . . . Oh my God, I thought, I'll never work
again. I'm old. But strangely enough, as I turn forty my gray
hairs and wrinkles don't bother me very much. I think it's because I'm happy. That always helps. And it's because I'm dis-
covering that if you work at it, and you're lucky, you really can
get wiser. I wouldn't want to go back."

Audrey Hepburn expressed something similar when she
emerged from a long retirement to take on a new movie role at
the age of forty-nine: "I don't mind in the least playing a woman
much younger than I am. Let the camera come in close. I've decided I like my wrinkles."

And at age seventy, Harold Child, editor of the *London
Times Literary Supplement,* told Margaret Sanger: "All the time

I was in my sixties I dreaded becoming seventy. But now that I am seventy, I don't mind it a bit."

POST MENOPAUSAL ZEST

Above all, remember that there is such a thing as PMZ, or Post Menopausal Zest.

Post Menopausal Zest means not only a renewed self-confidence but a renewed interest in living after a period of disruption.

The anthropologist Margaret Mead coined the phrase PMZ, and it kept her working and lecturing vigorously until she died at the age of seventy-six. And there is Martha Graham choreographing new dances at eighty-four, Alberta Hunter singing in cafes at eighty-six, and Louise Nevelson doing stunning big sculptures at eighty-two.

I could go on and on.

Somebody asked James J. Corbett, the world's heavyweight boxing champion, how one got to be a champion. He answered: "Get up from the mat after the count of nine and fight one more round."

Your adrenal hormones come to your rescue after the menopause and give you new strength and courage with which to fight on. Your PMZ can come to your rescue to give you a different kind of courage. Courage to change with the changing years.

So take your count of nine on the mat if you have to. Then be up and at life again—for that eternal one more round.

THE DOCTORS WHO HAVE HELPED ME
And Their Hospital Affiliations at the Time

DR. HENRY S. ACKEN, JR., Gynecology Consultant, Methodist Hospital, Brooklyn, New York.

DR. FRANK ADAIR, Chief, Breast Cancer Service, Memorial Hospital, New York.

DR. CELIA BERCOW, former Senior Physician, Brooklyn College.

DR. WILLIAM BICKERS, Gynecologist, Richmond, Virginia.

DR. CARL BINGER, Honorary Psychiatric Consultant, Harvard University Health Services, Cambridge, Massachusetts.

DR. CHARLES H. BIRNBERG, Attending Physician, Female Sex Endocrinology and Obstetrics, Brooklyn Jewish Hospital, Brooklyn, New York.

DR. IRVING BUNKIN, F.A.C.S., Diplomate, American Board of Obstetrics and Gynecology, New York.

DR. ALBERT M. CRANCE, F.A.C.S., Attending Urologist, Geneva General Hospital, Geneva, New York.

DR. HELENE DEUTSCH, Consultant Psychiatrist, Massachusetts General Hospital, Boston, Massachusetts.

DR. KONRAD DOBRINER, Sloan-Kettering Institute for Cancer Research, New York.

DR. HELEN FLANDERS DUNBAR, Associate Attending Psychiatrist, Columbia-Presbyterian Medical Center, New York.

DR. JOSEPH J. ELLER, Director, Department of Dermatology, New York City Hospital, New York.

DR. GEORGE FRIEDMAN, Professor of Clinical Medicine, Flower Fifth Ave Hospital, New York.

DR. ARTHUR GROLLMAN, Professor of Clinical Medicine, Southwestern Medical School, Dallas, Texas.

DR. ALAN F. GUTTMACHER, Chief, Department of Obstetrics and Gynecology, Mt. Sinai Hospital, New York.

DR. ROY HOSKINS, former Director of Research, Memorial Foundation of Neuro-endocrine Research, Harvard University, Cambridge, Massachusetts.

DR. RAPHAEL KURZROCK, PH.D., Consulting Endocrinologist, Morrisania City Hospital, New York.

DR. ALFRED A. LOESER, late Director, Gynecological and Obstetrical Department, Jewish Hospital, Berlin; Fellow of the Royal Academy of Medicine, London, England.

DR. THOMAS H. MCGAVACK, Professor of Clinical Medicine, New York Medical College, New York.

DR. WILLIAM I. MALAMUD, Professor of Psychiatry, Boston University, Boston, Massachusetts.

DR. EARLE MILLIARD MARSH, Medical Director, Institute for the Advanced Study of Human Sexuality, San Francisco, California.

DR. MARGARET MEAD, late Associate Curator, Museum of Natural History, New York, New York.

DR. EMY METZGER, Diplomate in Psychiatry, American Board of Neurology and Psychiatry, New York.

DR. JEAN BAKER MILLER, Psychiatrist, Boston, Massachusetts.

DR. EQUINN MUNNEL, Assistant Attending Obstetrician and Gynecologist, Columbia-Presbyterian Medical Center, New York.

DR. HERBERT POLLACK, Nutrition Committee, American Heart Association.

DR. ELEANOR PERCIVAL, Assistant Professor of Gynecology and Obstetrics, McGill University, Montreal, Canada.

DR. CLYDE L. RANDALL, Professor of Obstetrics and Gynecology, University of Buffalo Medical School, Buffalo, New York.

DR. JOHN STURDIVANT READ, Emeritus Professor of Urology, The College of Medicine at New York City, University of New York.

DR. ROBERT N. RUTHERFORD, Chief, Obstetrical Service, Virginia Mason Hospital, Seattle, Washington.

DR. UDALL J. SALMON, former Chief, Menopause and Gynecological Endocrine Clinic, Mt. Sinai Hospital, New York.

DR. LEWIS C. SCHEFFEY, Emeritus Professor of Obstetrics and Gynecology, Jefferson Medical School, Philadelphia, Pennsylvania.

DR. HANS SELYE, Professor of Medicine, Montreal University, Montreal, Canada.

DR. MARTIN SHEERER, Professor of Psychology, University of Kansas, Lawrence, Kansas.

DR. N. W. SHOCK, Chief, Section of Gerontology, National Heart Institute, National Institutes of Health and the Baltimore City Hospitals, Baltimore, Maryland.

DR. C. W. SHOPPEE, Professor of Internal Medicine, Swansea College, Swansea, Wales.

DR. EPHRAIM SHORR, Attending Physician, The New York Hospital, New York.

DR. EDWARD STIEGLITZ, Associate, Washington School of Psychiatry, Washington, D.C.

DR. ABRAHAM STONE, Director, Marriage Consultation Center, Community Church, New York, New York.

DR. SAMUEL TOPAL, Cooley-Dickinson Hospital, Northampton, Massachusetts.

DR. BERNARD A. WATSON, Clifton Springs Sanitarium and Clinic, Clifton Springs, New York.

DR. EDWARD WEISS, Professor of Clinical Medicine, Temple University Medical School, Philadelphia, Pennsylvania.

DR. LAWRENCE R. WHARTON, Professor of Obstetrics and Gynecology, Johns Hopkins University, Baltimore, Maryland.

Books and Articles That Have Helped Me

For General Background

GREENBLATT, ROBERT. *Office Endocrinology*. Charles C. Thomas, 1949.

GROLLMAN, ARTHUR. *Essentials of Endocrinology*. 2d ed. Lippincott, 1947.

HOSKINS, ROY. *The Tides of Life*. W. W. Norton, 1941.

KURZROCK, RAPHAEL. *The Endocrines in Obstetrics and Gynecology*. Williams and Wilkins, 1938.

RICCI, JAMES. *History of Gynecology*. Blakiston, 1943.

SCHEINFELD, AMRAM. *Women and Men*. Harcourt Brace, 1944.

SELYE, HANS. *Encyclopedia of Endocrinology*. A. W. T. Franks, Montreal, Canada, 1948.

SEWARD, GEORGENE. *Sex and the Social Order*. McGraw-Hill, 1946.

For Special Chapters

MENSTRUATION: A TIDE RISES AND FALLS

BENEDEK, THERESE, and RUBENSTEIN, BORIS P. "Psychological Corelation of Menstruation and Psycho-dynamic Processes." *Pyschosomatic Medicine,* 1:245, 1939.

CHADWICK, MARY. "Nervous and Mental Disease Monographs." No. 56, 1932.

FRAZER, SIR JAMES G. *The Golden Bough.* Macmillan, 1923.

HAMBLEN, E. C. *Female Sex Endocrinology.* Charles C. Thomas, 1938.

———. *Understanding Marriage and the Family.* Eugene Hugh, 1946.

MAILER, NORMAN. *Prisoner of Sex,* New American Library, 1971.

MILLS, C. A., and OGLE, C. "Physiologic Sterility of Adolescence." *Human Biology,* 8:607, 1936.

SUMNER, WILLIAM GRAHAM. *Folkways.* Ginn and Co., 1906.

THORN, NELSON and THORN. "The Mechanism of Edema Associated with Menstruation." *Endocrinology,* 22:165, 1938.

THOMPKINS and NEIBINGER. "Basal Body Temperature Graphs." *British Journal of Obstetrics and Gynecology,* 52:24, 1945.

THE WISDOM OF YOUR BODY

BICKERS, WILLIAM. *Outline of Clinical Gynecology,* 1948.

CANNON, WALTER. *The Wisdom of the Body.* W. W. Norton, 1932.

———. *Bodily Changes in Pain, Hunger, Fear and Rage.* W. W. Norton, 1929.

FLUHMANN, C. F. "Hormonal Relation of Menopausal Symptoms." *Journal of Clinical Endocrinology,* 4:12, 1944.

HAMBLEN, E. C. *Endocrinology of Women.* Charles C. Thomas, p. 23ff., 1945.

LOESER, A. A. "Male Hormones in Gynecology and Obstetrics." *Obstetrical and Gynecological Survey,* 3:363, 1948.

ROSS, R. A. "The Involutional Phase of the Menstrual Cycle," *American Journal of Obstetrics and Gynecology,* 45:497, 1943.

SHOPPEE, C. W. "Symposium on the Adrenal Cortex." *British Journal of Endocrinology,* 5:4, 1947.

How Your Doctor Can Help You

BICKERS, WILLIAM. "Post-menopausal Nocturia Treated with Testosterone." *Urologic and Cutaneous Review,* XLIX; 7, 1945.

BUXTON, C. L. "Medical Therapy during the Menopause." *Journal of Clinical Endocrinology,* 6:12, 1944.

CARTER, A. C., COHEN, I. J. and SHORR, E. "Androgens in Women." *Vitamins and Hormones,* 5:317, 1946.

DOHERTY, REKA. *Cancer.* Random House, 1950.

ELLER, J. J., and ELLER, W. D. "Cutaneous Effects of Topical Applications of Natural Estrogens." *Archives of Dermatology and Syphilology,* 59:499, 1949.

GEIST, S. H., and SALMON, U. J. "Are Estrogens Carcinogenic in the Human Female?" *American Journal of Obstetrics and Gynecology,* 41:1, 1941.

HAMBLEN, E. C. "Some Aspects of Sex Endocrinology in General Practice." *North Carolina Medical Journal,* 7:10, 1946.

LOESER, A. A. "Male Hormones in Gynecology and Obstetrics." *Obstetrical and Gynecological Survey,* June 1948.

NEUGARTEN, L., and STEINITZ, E. "Use of Estrogenic Suppositories in Vaginitis in Women." *Journal of Clinical Endocrinology,* 1:751, 1941.

NOVAK, E. "Some Misconceptions and Abuses in Gynecological Organo Therapy." *Pennsylvania Medical Journal,* 48:771, 1944.

PAPANICOLAOU, G. N., and SHORR, E. "Vaginal Smear." *American Journal of Obstetrics and Gynecology,* 31:806, 1936.

PAPANICOLAOU, G. N., and TROUT, H. F. "Diagnosis of Uterine Cancer by Vaginal Smear." *New York State Medical Journal,* 43:767, 1943.

PFEIFFER, C. A., and ALLEN, E. "Attempt to Produce Cancer in Rhesus Monkeys by Carcinogenic Hydrocarbons and Estrogens." *Cancer Research,* 8:3, 1943.

RUTHERFORD, ROBERT N. "Therapy during the Menopause—A Review." *Western Journal of Surgery and Gynecology,* 53:11, 1945.

SALMON, UDALL J. "Androgen Therapy in Gynecology." *Progress in Gynecology,* Grune & Stratton, 1946.

SEVRINGHAUS, E. L. "The Management of the Climacteric." Charles C. Thomas, 1948.

SEVRINGHAUS, E. L., and ST. JOHN, R. "Oral Use of Conjugated Estrogens—Equine." *Journal of Clinical Endocrinology,* 3:2, 1943.

SHORR, E. "The Menopause." *Bulletin of the Academy of Medicine,* 16:453, 1940.

———. "A New Technique for Staining Vaginal Smears." *Science,* 91:321 and 519, 1940.

STONER, W. H. "Use and Misuse of Hormones." *American Journal of Pharmacy,* 118:11, 1946.

WATSON, B. A. "Clinical Experiences with Oral Ethinyl Estradiol." *Journal of Clinical Endocrinology,* 7:447, 1942.

WERNER, A. A., and COLLIER, W. D. "The Effect of Theelin Injections on the Castrated Woman." *Journal of the American Medical Association,* 100:633, 1933.

HOW YOU CAN HELP YOURSELF

BRECHER, E. *Licit and Illicit Drugs.* Little Brown, 1972.

DEUTSCH, HELENE. *The Psychology of Women.* Grune and Stratton, Vol. II, p. 478, 1945.

JACKSON, JOSEPHINE A. and SALISBURY, HELEN. *Outwitting Our Nerves*. Appleton-Century-Crofts, pp. 60 and 125, 1944.

ROSS, T. A. *The Common Neuroses*. Edward Arnold & Co., London. 2d ed., p. 78, p. 143, 1937.

You Can Keep Your Sex Life

GREENBLATT, R. B. "Hormonal Factors in Libido," *Journal Clinical Endocrinology*, p. 305, 1943.

GUMPERT, MARTIN. *You Are Younger Than You Think*. Duell, Sloan and Pearce, p. 92, 1944.

HAMILTON, J. B. "Sex Activity in Eunuchs." *Anatomical Record*, 85:314, 1943.

LATZ, LEO. *The Rhythm of Sterility and Fertility in Women*. 6th revised ed. Latz Foundation, Chicago, pp. 110, 121ff., 1934.

LAWTON, GEORGE. *Aging Successfully*. Columbia University Press, pp. 126, 133, 1946.

LUND, FREDERICK. *Emotions of Men*. McGraw-Hill, p. 166, 1930.

REISS, MAX. "The Role of Sex Hormones in Psychiatry." *Journal of Mental Science*, 86:767, 1940.

TAUBER, E. S. "Effects of Castration on the Sexuality of the Adult Male." *Psychosomatic Medicine*, 2:74, 1940.

You Can Keep Your Figure

SCHMIDT, RUTH. Personal interview with the author.

You Can Keep Your Mind

COMFORT, ALEX. *A Good Age*. Crown Publishers, 1976.

FARRAR, C. B., and FRANK, RUTH. "Menopause and Psychosis." Paper read at 98th meeting of British Medical Association.

FLACH, FREDERIC. *Choices: Coping Creatively with Personal Change*. Lippincott, 1977.

FRIEZE, E. H., et al. *Women and Sex Roles.* W. W. Norton, 1978.

GRAY, MADELINE. *The Normal Woman.* Charles Scribner's Sons, 1971.

JAMIESON, G. R., and WALL, J. H. "Mental Reactions at the Climacterium." *American Journal of Psychiatry,* 11:901, 1932.

MALAMUD, WILLIAM I., and SANDS, S. L. "The Involutional Psychoses." *Psychosomatic Medicine,* Vol. III, No. IV, October 1941.

MILLER, JEAN BAKER. *Toward a New Psychology of Women.* Beacon Press, Boston, 1977.

Mental Health Statistics Current Reports. "Patients in State Mental Hospitals." MH-B50, No. 4, 1948.

ROSS, T. A. *The Common Neuroses,* 2d ed. Edward Arnold, London, p. 130, 1937.

STIEGLITZ, EDWARD. *The Second Forty Years.* Lippincott, 1946.

United States Public Health Service. *Mental Health in Late Maturity.* Supplement No. 168.

IS THERE A MALE CHANGE TOO?

ANDREWS, D. L. "A Simple Test for Hormone Deficiency in the Male," *Journal of Clinical Endocrinology,* 6:516, 1946.

BERGLER, EDMUND. "Some Recurrent Misconceptions Concerning Impotence." *Psychoanalytic Review,* 27:450, 1940.

DANIELS, G. E., and TAUBER, E. "A Dynamic Approach to Replacement Therapy in Castrates." *American Journal of Psychiatry,* 97:905, 1941.

GROLLMAN, ARTHUR. *Essentials of Endocrinology.* 2d ed. Lippincott, p. 485ff., 1947.

HECKEL, N. J. "Evaluation of Sex Hormones in Treatment of Diseases of the Genito-Urinary System." *Journal of Clinical Endocrinology,* 4:166, 1944.

HELLER, CARL G., and MADDOCK, WILLIAM. "The Use of Androgens in Men." *Bulletin of the New York Academy of Medicine,* 24:179, 1949.

HELLER, CARL G., and MYERS, GORDON B. "The Male Climacteric, Its Symptomology, Diagnosis, and Treatment." *Journal of the American Medical Association,* 126:472, 1944.

HEMMING, E. L. "The Truth About Testosterone." *Science Digest,* April 1946.

LISSER, H., and CURTIS, L. E. "Testosterone Therapy of Male Eunuchoids." *Journal of Clinical Endocrinology,* 3:388, 1943.

WERNER, A. A. "The Male Climacteric." *Journal of the American Medical Association,* 127:705, 1945.

LOVE AFTER FORTY, FIFTY, AND SIXTY

BUTLER, ROBERT N., and LEWIS, MYRNA I. *Sex After Sixty: A Guide for Men and Women for Their Later Years.* Harper & Row, 1976.

Einstein Story. New York *Times,* October 12, 1979.

Happiness Report. *Redbook* magazine, August 1978.

LEONARD, JOHN. "What Men Really Want From Women." *The Reader's Digest,* October 1979.

LEVINSON, DANIEL J., et al. *The Seasons of a Man's Life.* Alfred A. Knopf, 1978.

PLECK, JOSEPH H. and SAWYER, JACK, editors. *Men and Masculinity.* Prentice-Hall, 1974.

POMEROY, WARDELL B. "Don't Let These Myths Undermine Your Sex Life." *The Reader's Digest,* October 1979.

STEWART, WENDY. "A psychological study of the formation of the early adult life structure in women." Dissertation, Columbia University, 1977.

ZILBERGELD, BERNIE. *Male Sexuality: A Guide to Sexual Fulfillment.* Little Brown, 1978.

THE ESTROGEN-CANCER SCARE

"Behind the Estrogen Cancer Debate." *Medical World News,* October 4, 1976.

"Estrogen May Raise CA Risk in Some Patients." *Ob/Gyn. News,* June 15, 1977.

"Estrogens and Cancer of the Endometrium." *Southern Medical Journal,* January 1977.

"Estrogens and Endometrial Cancer." Department of Health, Education, and Welfare Drug Bulletin, February–March 1976.

Estrovis, Patient Trial Pack. Parke-Davis Laboratories, February 10, 1980.

"Exogenous Estrogen, Endometrial Cancer Link Questioned." *Ob/Gyn. News,* June 15, 1975.

GREENBLATT, ROBERT B. "Must the Alleged Link Between Estrogens and Cancer Change the Way You Treat Menopausal Patients?" *Modern Medicine,* March 1, 1977.

JONES, S. GEORGEANNA, and ROSS, WALTER S. "Estrogen and Cancer," *Reader's Digest,* November 1978.

KUPPERMAN, HERBERT S. "The Beneficial Effects of Estrogen." *The Female Patient,* February 1980.

NOVAK, EDMUND R., and WOODRUFF, RONALD J., *Obstetric and Gynecologic Pathology,* 7th ed., Saunders, 1974.

PECK, RICHARD L. "The Estrogen-Cancer Flap: What You Need to Know." *Current Prescribing,* Special Report, May 1976.

ROSENFELD, ALBERT. "Skin Exposed." *Saturday Review,* July 22, 1978.

SMITH, DONALD C., et al. "Association of Exogenous Estrogen and Endometrial Carcinoma." *New England Journal of Medicine,* December 4, 1975.

"Testimony on Estrogen-Replacement is Conflicting." *Ob/Gyn. News,* January 15, 1976.

"What You Should Know About Estrogens." *Patient Package Insert,* Ayerst Laboratories, Inc., September 20, 1977.

Go Easy on Hysterectomy

DOYLE, J. C. "Unnecessary Ovariectomies." *Journal of the American Medical Association,* 148:1105, 1952.

———. "Unnecessary Hysterectomies." *Journal of the American Medical Association,* 151:360, 1953.

ENGLISH, O. SPURGEON, and PEARSON, GERALD H. *Emotional Problems of Living.* W. W. Norton, p. 362, 1945.

KINSEY, ALFRED C. *Sexual Behavior in the Human Male.* W. B. Saunders, p. 576, 1945.

MILLER, NORMAN. "Hysterectomy: Medical Necessity or Surgical Racket?" *Journal of Obstetrics and Gynecology,* 51:804, 1946.

NUGENT, NANCY. *Hysterectomy.* Doubleday, Garden City, New York, 1976.

RANDALL, CLYDE L. "Ovarian Function After the Menopause." *Journal of Obstetrics and Gynecology,* 74:4, 1957.

RAY, MARIE BENYON, *How Never to Be Tired.* Bobbs-Merrill, p. 202, 1938, 1944.

LOOKING FORWARD

COMFORT, ALEX. *A Good Age.* Crown Publishers, New York, 1976.

FEINSTEIN, HERBERT, and BAER, JEAN. *Stop Running Scared.* Dell, 1977.

LESHAN, EDA. *The Wonderful Crisis of Middle Age.* Warner Paperback Library, 1974.

ADDITIONAL ACKNOWLEDGMENTS

Additional thanks to the publishers who have given me permission to quote from these articles and books:

The Psychology of Women. Vol. II. Helene Deutsch. Grune and Stratton, Inc., 1945.

The Emotions of Men. Frederick Lund. McGraw-Hill Book Company, Inc., 1930.

Peace of Soul. Fulton J. Sheen. McGraw-Hill Book Company, Inc., 1954.

"Use and Misuse of Hormones." W. H. Stoner. *American Journal of Pharmacy,* 1946.

The Rhythm of Sterility and Fertility in Women. 6th revised ed. Latz Foundation, 1934.

The Emotional Problems of Living. English and Pearson. W. W. Norton and Company, Inc., 1945.

The Endocrinology of Women. E. C. Hamblen. Charles C. Thomas, 1945.

"An Attempt to Produce Cancer in Rhesus Monkeys by Carcinogenic Hydrocarbons and Estrogens." Pfeiffer and Allen. *Cancer Research,* 1945.

Aging Successfully. George Lawton. Columbia University Press, 1946.

Sexual Behavior in the Human Male. Alfred C. Kinsey. W. B. Saunders Company, 1948.

The Common Neuroses. T. A. Ross. Edward Arnold Co., 1937.

Estrogen and Cancer. S. Georgeanna Jones, *The Reader's Digest,* November 1978.

Index

Acne, 54–55
  androgen hormone treatment and,
    82–83
Adair, Dr. Frank, 83
Adolescence, 8–9, 170
  androgen hormone treatment for
    boys, 53–54
  the pituitary gland and, 18
Adolescent acne, 54–55
Adrenal glands, 15–18, 19, 227
  androgen and, 57, 65, 115
  estrogen and, 57, 65
  menopause and, 65
Adrenal hormones, 17, 59–60, 87,
  249
Ageless Woman, The (Kaufman),
  89–90
Aging
  cellular therapy for, 89–90
  myths about, 245–46
  retardation of, 89–91
Aging Successfully (Lawton), 127
Alcohol, 146
  as a stimulant, 201
Alimony, 174
Alvarez, Dr. Walter C., 230
American Gynecological Society,
  226
American Heart Association, 150
American Pharmaceutical
  Association, 83
Androgen, 50–57, 70, 115, 227
  adrenal glands and, 57, 65, 115
  body fat and, 55

effect on skin and hair, 54–55
  homosexuality and, 55–56
  presence in women, 51–53, 56, 57
  sex drive and, 54, 56
  source of, 56–57
  strength and, 53
Androgen hormone treatment
  for adolescent boys, 53–54
  after hysterectomy, 53
  for males, 181–84
  as menopausal medicine, 81–83
    harmful effects of overdosage,
      82–83
  the pituitary gland and, 181, 183
Anesthesia, 4–5
Anger, 175–76
Animals
  periods of "heat" in, 110–11
  sexual activity in, 119–20
Animal urine as natural source of
  estrogen, 78–79
Anxiety, 92
  self-help for, 95–98
Aptitude tests, 104
Arey, Dr. L. B., 44
Aristotle, 176
Arteriosclerosis, 227–28
Artificial birth-control methods,
  122, 124
Atrophic vaginitis, 213
Augustine, St., 123
Aureomycin, 244
Ayer's Cherry Pectoral, 169